HEALTH FROM GOD'S GARDEN

A renowned herbalist with many years
experience in treating people suffering from
both minor complaints and serious
illnesses sets out everything she knows
about herbs and herbal remedies.

HEALTH FROM GOD'S GARDEN

Herbal Remedies for Glowing Health and Glorious Well~Being

Maria Treben

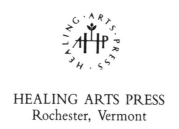

HEALING ARTS PRESS
Rochester, Vermont

Healing Arts Press
One Park Street
Rochester, Vermont 05767
www.InnerTraditions.com

Healing Arts Press is a division of Inner Traditions International

Note to the reader: *This book is intended as an informational guide. The remedies, approaches, and techniques described herein are meant to supplement, and not to be a substitute for, professional medical care or treatment. They should not be used to treat a serious ailment without prior consultation with a qualified health care professional.*

Library of Cangress Cataloging-in-Publication Data
Treben, Maria.
[Heilkraüter aus dem Garten Gottes. English]
Health from God's garden: herbal remedies for glowing health
and welpbeing / Maria Treben.
p.   cm.
Translation of: Heilkraüter aus dem Garten Gottes.
Includes indexes.
ISBN 978-0-89281-235-6
1. Material medica, Vegetable. 2. Medicine—Formulae, recipes, prescriptions.
3. Therapeutics—Popular works. I. Title.
RS164.T 7813 1988
615′.321—dc19   88-23541

Printed and bound in India

26

About the Author

Maria Treben gave her first informal talk on the medicinal value of plants in 1971, and the interest that this generated was so great that it turned what was a hobby into a full-time occupation.

In the following years her popularity grew rapidly and, in addition to lecturing throughout Austria and West Germany, she wrote a book entitled Health from God's Pharmacy *which was published in 1980. This title became a number-one bestseller overnight— sales now totalling over four million copies with editions in seven different languages.*

Maria Treben garnered respect all over the world as a leading authority on medicinal herbs. In this new, more extensive and exhaustive book she details everything she learned from her long experience in using herbal remedies for treating a wide range of ailments.

Contents

Publisher's Note

Maria Treben uses metric measures to express the quantities of the constituents of her herbal remedies. For the convenience of the reader we have added approximate imperial equivalents. These have been rounded to the nearest half ounce, which results in apparent anomalies such as 1 oz being shown for both 25g and 30g. The difference is so small, however, that it will not affect the remedy.

Introduction

Nearly ten years have passed since the publication of my first book, *Health from God's Pharmacy*. The book's success was phenomenal, and this is something that both delighted and overwhelmed me. On the one hand it meant that my knowledge about the medicinal herbs to be found in God's garden and their wonderful healing properties was being made available to many people and that had been my deepest and most heartfelt wish when I wrote the book. On the other hand the book's publication, and especially its unexpected success, was in many ways a very mixed blessing, changing my life beyond recognition and creating a great many unexpected difficulties for both me and my family.

I would like to take this opportunity to make it very, very clear that I would never ever advise anyone to dispense with their doctor's diagnosis, help and advice. Anyone who did this would be endangering their own health unnecessarily, and I am interested in helping people to regain their health, not to endanger it. So please, do trust your doctor — your health is his job. And above all, tell him what you are doing if you decide to use any of the herbs and recipes described in this book. He needs to know this in order to be able to treat you properly.

Unfortunately there are still some traditional doctors of the old school who may stubbornly refuse to condone the use of herbs. Such an attitude can destroy the mutual trust of physician and patient. Even so, the reason for their refusal is not ill will, it is simply that they are not willing to be open to anything which they do not understand; even the most self-evident healing successes are not enough to convince them so long as they are unable to explain why the herbs work. In a way, I am in the same position as them — I know that the herbs work and how to use them effectively, but I do not know why they work. The difference is that I am perfectly happy to accept these gifts of God without knowing the whys and hows.

It is gratifying that some chemical and pharmaceutical companies are researching in the field of herbal medicine and that they are now devoting some of their money and energy to finding out why medicinal herbs are so effective. For some time our ever-increasing dependence on artificial fertilizers and all the other products of the chemical industry has been polluting our food and drink and causing new illnesses which we then try to treat with yet more chemicals. And we have not only been damaging ourselves but also passing on all these illnesses to our children. The revival of interest in herbal medicine is part of the trend toward tackling those problems.

This is one of the main reasons for my deciding to write this new book, for I am more convinced than ever of the value of herbal medicine. I have learned a great deal more about medicinal herbs over the last ten years. I have attended countless lectures and seminars dealing with all aspects of herbal medicine and the problems involved; I have become aquainted with many new herbs and their uses; and above all thousands of letters from readers of my first book have confirmed the value of my suggestions and recipes again and again. This book is the tangible result of all this experience.

I have done my best to write a practical handbook for the entire family, a book that is easy to understand and easy to use. The contents are organized alphabetically. When you look up the illness in question you will find all the relevant herbal recipes and treatments, together with instructions for their preparation and use.

In closing I do have one request: I have made every effort to make this book as complete and as comprehensive as possible. Please don't visit me or telephone me or ask me to send you herbs or additional recipes. All you need to do is to read the book — it contains everything I know!

How to Use This Book

The information in this book is organized alphabetically, so there is no need for a detailed index. Simply look up the illness which you wish to treat and you will find everything you need to know. To make finding the right information even easier the book has also been subdivided into the following sections.

1. The Medicinal Herbs in God's Garden   page 17

An alphabetical list of the medicinal herbs used in this book, together with colour illustrations and information about where they grow and when they are most potent. In addition this chapter also contains a number of practical tips for collecting, drying and storing medicinal herbs.

2. Prevention is Better than a Cure   page 33

This chapter contains descriptions of all the herbal teas and other recipes which can be used as preventive remedies, to help purify the body and strengthen its resistance to illness and disease.

3. The Gentle Way to Health   page 36

Here you will find all the illnesses and complaints that can be treated with the help of simple home remedies.

4. Faith Can Move Mountains page 83

This chapter covers the treatment of the more serious illnesses. It is *absolutely essential* that a qualified physician be consulted before you attempt to treat these diseases.

5. Standard Herbal Recipes   page 118

Under the headings in the two main chapters containing the lists of the various individual illnesses you will find all the medicinal herbs that can be used to treat the illness in question, together with instructions on how to use them. In many cases several different herbal teas are listed, and so long as no specific instructions are given regarding the order in which they should be taken, you can select the tea that agrees with you best or which you can obtain most easily.

For convenience, standard recipes for several teas, tinctures, ointments, etc., have been grouped here in alphabetical order. If you need the recipe for a treatment which is marked with an asterisk in Chapters 2, 3 and 4, simply refer to this section, following the instructions for the recipe's use given under the appropriate ailment heading in the preceding chapters.

Identifying Medicinal Herbs

The simple act of going out into the country to look for medicinal herbs is in itself a great boon to our health, for it takes us away from the hustle and bustle of the towns and cities and into the quiet and freedom of nature. If you try it, you will soon see for yourself how good these long, relaxed walks are for your body, for they fulfill a very deep and basic human need.

If you have no previous experience with medicinal herbs it is a good idea at first to concentrate on getting to know the countryside, looking in the places where the herbs are most likely to be found and learning to identify them in their natural environment. And if you do not yet feel confident about being able to identify the plants on your own you can take part in guided walks and outings organized by nature clubs and other groups under the guidance of experts in order to gain the necessary knowledge. The danger of gathering poisonous plants by accident is not so great in the case of the herbs dealt with in this book (mushrooms are much more risky!) — on the contrary, it is much more likely that someone who doesn't know what they are doing will do unnecessary damage to the environment. Many medicinal herbs are endangered and protected species,* and there are some useless herbs that look very similar to their medicinal cousins; it would be a pity and a waste to pick them unnecessarily. So please do make sure that you know enough to be able to identify the plants you really need before you set off to collect them.

Collecting Herbs

Fresh herbs, which, medicinally speaking, are more potent than the dried variety, can be gathered from early spring through late autumn. Some herbs, such as the great plantain, bedstraw and celandine can even be found growing in the wild in winter, if it is mild enough.

If possible it is advisable to pick the herbs on a sunny day; apart from the fact that it is more enjoyable, the medicinal potency of the herbs picked when the sun is shining is considerably higher. It is also important to take care to pick the

* The Endangered Species Act actually makes the taking of certain wild plants illegal.

herbs as far away from polluted areas, busy roads and industrial installations as possible. The plants should be cut off at least two finger-breadths above the ground; never ever pull them out by the roots! A wicker basket is the best container for carrying your freshly-picked herbs home (plastic bags should be avoided at all costs). And, finally, please do take care not to collect more herbs than you really need!

Storing and Drying Herbs

Whenever possible, medicinal herbs should be used while they are still fresh. Any extra herbs left over (and this should be as small a quantity as possible) can be stored for later use. In order to prepare them for storage first chop them up finely and then lay them out to dry in a shady and airy spot, on clean cloths or sheets of wrapping paper. The herbs shouldn't be washed before they are laid out to dry — this is why it is important to pick them in a clean, unpolluted place. Once they are really dry they can then be stored in cardboard boxes, paper bags or dark-coloured glass jars. Tin cans and plastic containers or plastic bags should never be used for storing herbs. Dried herbs used for making teas can be kept for as long as a year, and any left over after this time can still be used for making herbal baths.

Important Note:

If the recipes, teas, tinctures and baths described in this book don't seem to be working for you, it is a good idea to engage the services of a dowser who can check your home and your place of work for geopathic fields. He will then be able to find places free of these negative vibrations so that you can change the position of your bed or desk, etc, and thus avoid exposing yourself to them.

HERB FARMS

Blue Sage Herb Farm, 406 Post Oak Road, Fredricksburg, Texas, 78624. (512) 997-6529. Plants and dried herbs.

Cedarbrook Herb Farm, 986 Sequim Avenue South, Sequim, Washington, 98382. (206) 683-7733. Plants.

Meadowbrook Herb Garden, Route 138, Wyoming, Rhode Island, 02898. (401) 539-7603. A biodynamic, organic farm. Plants, seeds, dried herbs.

Taylor's Herb Gardens, 1535 Lone Oak Road, Vista, California, 92084. (619) 727-3485. Plants and seeds.

Well Sweep Herb Farm, 317 Mount Bethel Road, Port Murray, New Jersey, 07865. (201) 852-5390. Plants. Mail order available.

Woodland Herb Farm, Route 1, Box 105, Northport, Michigan, 49670. (616) 386-5081. Plants and dried herbs.

DRIED HERB SUPPLIERS

Aphrodisia Products, Inc., 282 Bleeker Street, New York, New York, 10014. (212) 989-6440. 200 varieties. Mail order available.

Dragon's Herbarium, 4642 SW Beaverton Hillsdale Highway, Portland, Oregon, 97221. (503) 244-7049. 250 varieties. Personal shoppers only.

Harvest Health Inc., 1944 Eastern Avenue SE, Grand Rapids, Michigan, 49507. (616) 245-6268. Mail order available.

The Herb Company, 206 West Maple, Independence, Missouri, 64050. (816) 254-9970. 300 varieties. Mail order available.

Indiana Botanic Gardens, Inc., P.O. Box 5, Hammond, Indiana, 46325. (219) 931-2480. 500 varieties. Mail order available.

Nature's Herb Company, 281 Ellis Street, San Francisco, California, 94102. (415) 474-2756. 200 varieties. Mail order available.

Penn Herb Company, 603 North 2nd Street, Philadelphia, Pennsylvania, 19123. (215) 925-3336. 700 varieties. Mail order available.

FORMULA SOURCES

Some formulas described in *Health from God's Garden* may be obtained through Nature Works, 5310 Derry Avenue, Suite H, Agoura, California, 91301. (818) 889-1602.

In Canada, Maria Treben's formulas may be obtained through Flora Distributors Ltd., 7400 Fraser Park Drive, Burnaby, British Columbia, V5J 5B9. (604) 438-1133.

Letters to the Author

In the ten years since the publication of my first book I have received a great many heartening letters from people who have managed to treat themselves successfully with the help of herbal remedies from God's garden. Below you will find a few excerpts from some of these letters, which I include here as a demonstration of the sort of thing that is possible when faith and herbal medicine work hand in hand.

I am sure that my critics will be very quick to object, saying that these are statements made by laymen, that they have no scientific value and that they don't, prove anything. To be perfectly frank, this doesn't bother me in the least. I know that the men and women who wrote these letters are ordinary, simple people, but what is wrong with that? In my opinion their letters are a precious source of hope and inspiration. The proof of the pudding is in the eating, and these letters are testaments to something that I feel is very important, no matter whether it is scientifically valid or not.

In the introduction to this book I made a point of asking you not to write to me. I would like to make it very clear, however, that this request only applies to letters asking for advice — I am always delighted to receive letters telling me about your experiences with my recipes and suggestions. As far as requests for advice are concerned, I can only repeat what I said in the introduction: please *don't* write asking me for advice; everything I know can be found in this book, and if you look for it you will find it!

(The writers of the following letters have asked me to respect their privacy, and it is thus not possible to publish their names and addresses here.)

I attended your lecture in Schwäbisch Hall, and I must say that I admire and respect you very much. I had a myoma, and I managed to get rid of it with the help of yarrow baths. When I showed the results to my doctor he was very surprised, and said that he couldn't understand it. God bless you and protect you.

The pain in my knees and other joints was so intense that I could no longer walk or climb the stairs. I was in such despair that I used to cry all the time. In the hospital they gave me injections for the pain. The doctor said that I had periostitis, so I made myself some comfrey root tincture and applied comfrey poultices to the painful joints while I was waiting for the tincture to be ready. I felt better straight away. Ten days later I started massaging the joints with the comfrey root tincture six or seven times a day, and I also took care to keep them very warm. The pain was gone within eight days. It's a miracle, I can hardly believe it.

I had already had two major operations, without any success. The Swedish bitters cured my gall-bladder disease. The doctors were very surprised, but I didn't tell them what it was that had cured me.

I started taking teas made with shepherd's purse and calamus root and two weeks later the intestinal hemorrhages started to get better. I hardly know how to tell you how much this means to me. The doctors tried to help me for a whole year without any success. I had felt very depressed throughout that time and had given up all hope of getting better. Now, thanks to you, my life has become worth living again! God bless you, and your work!

My brother's brother-in-law had cirrhosis of the liver, and the doctors at the hospital told him that it was incurable and sent him home. He started to drink club moss tea regularly and his health has been good for four years now.

I had a chronic bladder infection which didn't seem to be getting any better for six months, despite the doctor's treatment. What finally cured me was tea made from the small-flowered willow-herb, which I picked fresh every day.

My brother couldn't eat any longer. The doctors operated and for a while it seemed as though everything was all right again, but then he had a serious setback and had to go into hospital again. In hospital they told him that he had cancer of the pancreas and that there were already a great many metastases. Everybody feared the worst. He started to drink bedstraw tea every day, and the improvement was immediate. The metastases disappeared and my brother is now in good health once again. Everybody is talking about this wonderful cure. Thank you very much for your help.

When I returned home from hospital after an operation I suddenly became so hoarse that I couldn't speak at all. The doctors told me that my vocal cords were paralysed on the left side. I gargled with bedstraw and mallow tea every day and applied Swedish bitters compresses to my throat at night. I am so happy that I can talk again. I don't think there is any way that I can express my gratitude to God for this blessing.

I had breast cancer. After two operations I began a course of radiation treatment. It was hell on earth. One year later my other breast had to be removed as well, because the doctors had failed to notice a lump in it. It was an indescribable nightmare. The results of the tests went from bad to worse, and I felt completely drunk and dizzy all the time from the radiation treatment. I don't think there is any way I can describe just how depressed and hopeless I felt. But then the young director of our firm told me how he had cured himself of cancer of the spine with herbs, and I started to drink yarrow, calendula and nettle tea every day, along with six mouthfuls of the calamus root tea. Now I feel fine and my blood counts couldn't be better. All I can say is thank you, thank you.

I suffered from a constriction of the cystic duct for many years, and I took all sorts of different medicines, but the only thing that has really helped has been the Swedish bitters. It is nothing short of a miracle.

I had a severe case of chronic bronchitis that had lasted for a year and a half. The doctors gave me cortisone and all sorts of other injections, but they brought me only temporary relief. I was in great despair. My mother died of a similar asthmatic disease, after many years of illness. I am a very realistic person, and I was very sceptical at first. Even so, I started taking the plantain and thyme teas, and the club moss tea as well, and I started to get better a week later. Now, seven weeks later, I can go back to work again. I can even take part in sports again and go hiking. My life has become enjoyable again. My family and all my friends are very happy. We have come to understand that nature can give us very wonderful things, even though we still don't want to underestimate the value of the doctors' diagnosis, which as you rightly say is very important.

I went to one gynecologist after another for years on end. I had a terrible discharge. The last doctor I went to suggested having a hysterectomy, since the pills and suppositories didn't seem to be helping at all. Instead I started drinking a cup of yarrow tea every day (I picked the yarrow myself while the sun was shining) and six weeks later I was cured of this unpleasant condition.

My little granddaughter caught her heel in the spokes of her bicycle. It was a very nasty wound. I applied comfrey ointment to the wound and now her heel is better and the proud flesh has almost disappeared. She's so happy that she can run and jump and play again.

My husband had a sore on one of his toes caused by a shoe that was too small for him, and I applied some fresh ribwort leaf juice to the wound. It healed very quickly, even though his toes had been frostbitten while he was in Russia. It is wonderful to be able to avoid all the side-effects caused by chemical medicines.

1. The Medicinal Herbs in God's Garden

Agrimony
Agrimonia eupatoria

This popular medicinal plant is a member of the rose family. It grows in sunny, barren spots, usually in loamy soil, on embankments, at the edges of woods and forests, in ruins, pastures, open woods and rough meadows. The plant reaches a height of around 3 ft (90cm). The small yellow flowers with their central red patch grow on the stem. The toothed leaves are covered with coarse hairs and are dark green on the upper surface and a lighter green underneath. Agrimony blooms from the middle through late summer. The entire plant has medicinal properties, and it should be picked before it sets seed. The plants should be cut off cleanly above the ground and then chopped up finely and laid out to dry in thin layers. Agrimony has a pungent, spicy aroma and tastes a little bitter. You can tell whether the plants are good or not when you dry them: the blooms and leaves of medically potent agrimony will retain their colour when they are dried.

Arnica
Arnica montana

A flower-bearing stem, which reaches a length of between 12 and 20 in (30-50cm), grows out of a rosette of short, slightly hairy leaves resting on the ground. Two more flower-bearing stems with slightly smaller flowers grow out of the two leaves on the main stem. The petals of the yellowish-orange flowers have a covering of very fine silky hair, and they have a pleasantly fragrant aroma. Arnica can still be found in untouched mountainous regions, in forest glades and meadows, and also in peat bogs and damp, marshy meadows. These are the places that the farmers leave untouched when they mow the hay. Grazing animals avoid this plant. Arnica cannot survive on meadows that have been sprayed with artificial fertilizer. One farmer told me that the area where he lives used to be full of arnica before the introduction of artificial fertilizer, but that now he cannot find a single arnica blossom anywhere.

The inexperienced often confuse arnica with goatsbeard (or Jack-go-to-bed-at-noon), as both plants have similar, dark-yellow blossoms. The differences are as follows: arnica blossoms are darker yellow than those of the goatsbeard; the outer coating of the sepaloid leaves is covered with soft hair; and the blossoms are incomparably more fragrant. Arnica blossoms contain *arnicin* (an amaroid), essential oils, resin and tannin. The plant blossoms in early summer through midsummer, and into late summer in cooler climates. Arnica is most commonly found on the sunny sides of meadows.

It is found in sunny parts of meadows and woods. The floral calyces often contain the little black eggs of the cherry fruit-fly. A farmer from my home district in the Sudentenland once told me that these fruit flies protect the grain crops from pests and ergot. Be that as it may, these eggs must be removed by steeping the flower petals in alcohol before they are prepared for use.

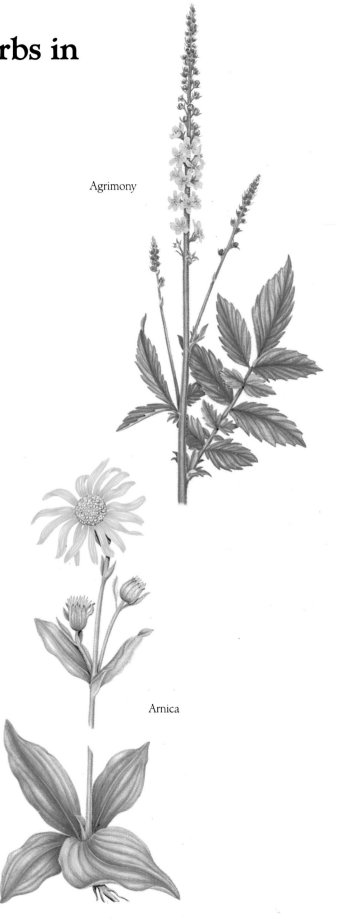

Agrimony

Arnica

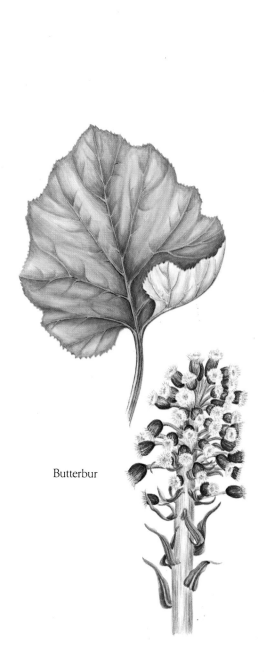

Butterbur

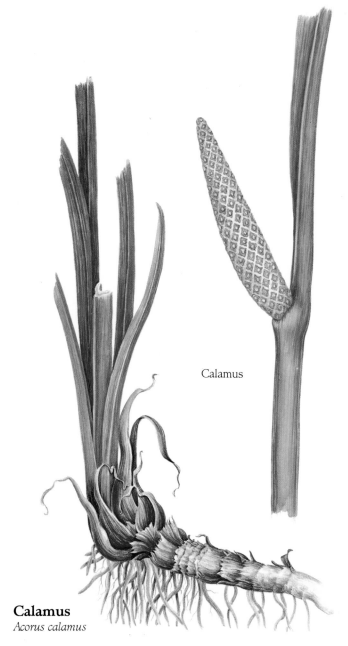

Calamus

Calamus
Acorus calamus

Calamus, or sweet flag, is a reedy water plant that grows in ponds, still waterways, lakes and also in perennially damp, swampy ground. The roots of the plant grow underwater; they are white, and when they are fresh they are as thick as your thumb and up to 3½ ft (100cm) long. These roots have a distinctive scent, giving the impression that they contain substances that have an invigorating effect on the nerves. Sword-shaped leaves, which can reach heights of up to 4 ft (120cm), grow up out of the root and resemble those of reeds or irises. Curved, brownish-yellow cobs appear on the green stalk of the plant in midsummer.

The only part of the plant that is of any medicinal value is the root, which should be dug up in the spring or autumn. After being cleaned and freed of any offshoots, the roots are prepared for use by dicing them finely and drying them. Calamus contains aromatic bitters and is a good stomach remedy. In Germany it is also known as German ginger, and people used to preserve the roots in the same way as real ginger. A powdered root extract can be used as a bath essence for the treatment of some illnesses. Calamus is a hardy plant.

Butterbur
Petasites officinalis

The butterbur grows along the banks of rivers and streams and on the edges of woods and forests. It is a spring plant, and the reddish-yellow flowers appear before the leaves. The leaves are furry on the undersides and can grow to the size of a broad-brimmed hat; in fact, in the past people used them as sunshades when the sun was too hot. They contain substances that, when applied as compresses, are excellent for alleviating the pain caused by sprains and dislocated joints. The roots should be collected before the flowers appear as they begin to lose their potency at this stage.

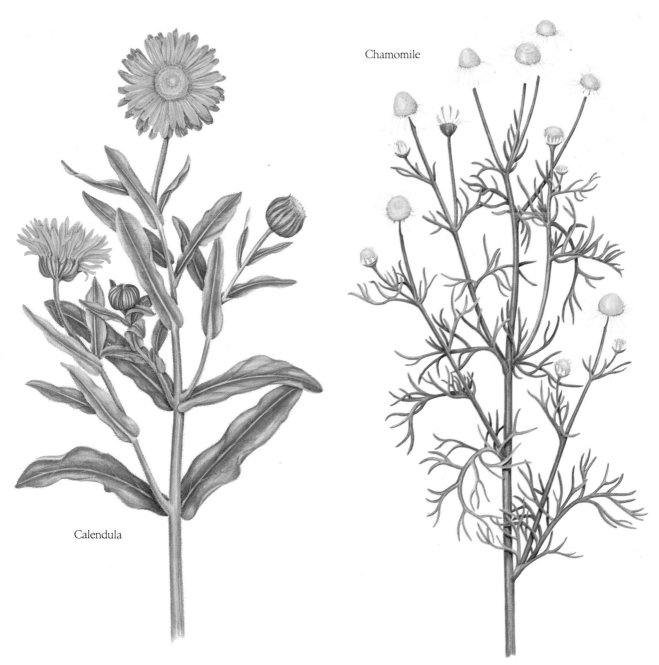

Chamomile

Calendula

Calendula
Calendula officinalis

Calendula, or pot marigold, is another member of the aster family. It is often used as a garden plant, but it can also be found growing wild in sheltered copses and around rubbish dumps. The plant reaches a height of around 2 ft (60cm) and has thick, fleshy, very juicy stems and longish, undivided leaves covered with fine hair. The flowers, which range in colour from bright yellow to dark orange, exude a very unusual, pungent fragrance in sunshine. The surface of calendula plants feels a little sticky and oily.

According to an old folk tradition the weather can be predicted accurately by watching calendula flowers: country folk say that the flowers never open in the morning if rain is on the way, but if they do open up before 7 a.m., you can be sure of fine weather.

Chamomile
Matricaria chamomille

Wild chamomile is a member of the aster family. It grows in fields (especially in corn, potato and beet fields), along country paths, among rubble and on fallow land. It is particularly fond of loamy soil. Chamomile has branched stalks and small, feathery leaves, reaches a height of around 20 in (50cm), and blooms from July to September. The yellow centre of the flower is hollow, a feature that distinguishes genuine medicinal chamomile from other varieties. It's best to pick the flowers at midday when the sun is shining as their essential oils are much more potent at this time. The aromatic fragrance of chamomile flowers is very soothing. The true chamomile should not be confused with the common chamomile that can be found in many private gardens.

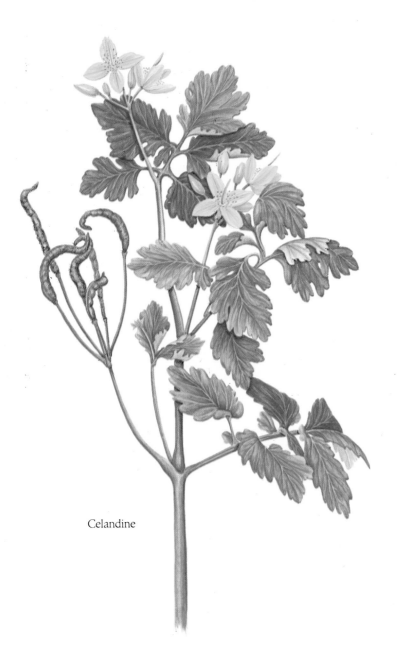

Celandine

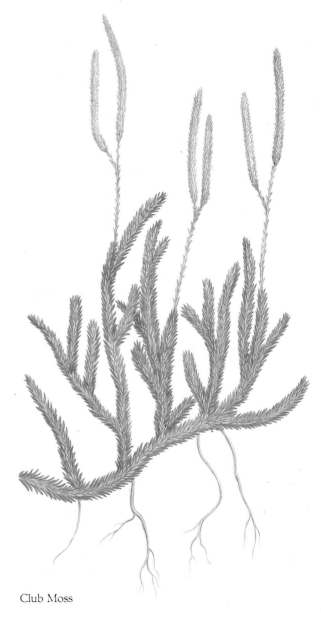

Club Moss

Celandine
Chelidonium majus

Celandine grows in sunny areas in hedgerows, along walls and fences, and at the edges of woods and forests. The rootstock is yellowish-orange, and the branched stalk, which contains a yellowish-orange sap, can reach heights of up to around 30 in (80cm). The shape of the leaves is similar to that of oak leaves. Celandine starts to flower in late spring and, if you cut off the seedpods (it often grows in gardens) when the flowers wither, the plant will continue to flower throughout the summer. The color of the four-petalled flowers ranges from bright yellow to a yellowish-orange. The roots should be collected in the spring and the autumn, and the plant itself while it is in blossom (more or less the whole summer). Many writers on herbal medicine (especially the medieval herbalist Tabernaemontanus) mention the fact that swallows pluck off little pieces of celandine leaf and rub the unopened eyes of their young with them — an indication of the value of this plant in the treatment of eye diseases. As a result, in some parts of Europe it is referred to as eye-herb or swallow-herb.

Club Moss
Lycopodium clavatum

This pteriodophyte plant resembles some varieties of moss. Its runners grow along the surface of the ground; they reach lengths of between 40 and 60 in (100-150cm) and are covered with soft, needle-shaped leaves. Starting in late summer the branches bear spadices that are between 4 and 6 in (10-15cm) long and that contain the plant's spores. Club moss can be picked from spring through fall, and the spores can be collected in early fall. It can also be found in dry, evergreen forests in upland areas at least 700m above sea level, but more commonly it grows in acid, sandy soil on northern mountain slopes and in mountain forests, both among the trees and at the edge of the woods.

20

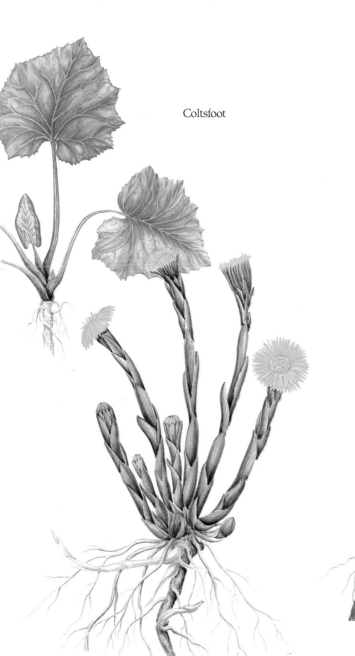

Coltsfoot

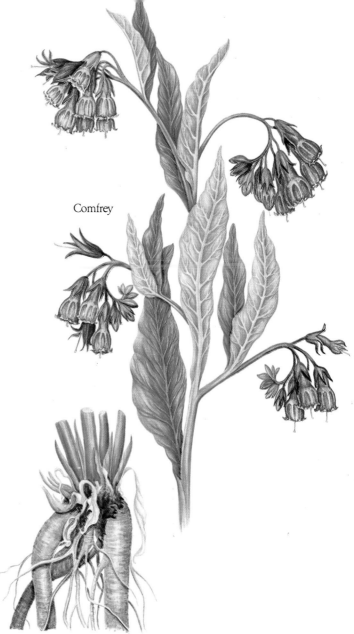

Comfrey

Coltsfoot
Tussilago farfara

This plant gets its name from the shape of its leaves, which resembles the imprint of a colt's hoof on the ground. The coltsfoot is a member of the aster family. Its golden-yellow flowers appear early in the year. The plant is commonly found in loamy soil, in sand and gravel pits, and along country paths and the edges of fields. The calyces stay open while the sun is shining and close again as soon as the sky clouds over. The leaves are silvery on the underside and appear between three and four weeks after the flowers. The rootstock is large, with many branches. The scaly stems bearing the golden-yellow blooms appear in the first days of spring. The flowers are similar to those of a dandelion but are considerably smaller. Coltsfoot leaves are very similar to butterbur leaves, so it is important to take care to identify the plant properly. In antiquity the coltsfoot was greatly prized as a remedy for coughs and lung infections, and doctors used to tell their patients to smoke the dried leaves in pipes, like tobacco.

Comfrey
Symphytum officinale

Comfrey grows in damp fields and meadows, in ditches, in damp fallow land, along the banks of streams, irrigation trenches and ponds, and at the edges of woods. Mature comfrey plants reach a height of about 2 ft (60cm). The coarse, hairy stems grow out of a rosette of leaves. These lance-shaped, light-green leaves, which can reach lengths of up to about 6 in (15cm), are coarse, hairy and have pointed tips. The roots can be a good 1½ in (4cm) thick, and they reach about 1 ft (30cm) down into the ground. They are brittle, breaking amazingly easily, and very slimy and greasy to the touch. The roots can be dug out of the ground in the spring or autumn. The colour of the bell-shaped blossoms, which hang down as though they were examining the ground below them, ranges from pink to light-blue to yellowish to white. Comfrey flowers in early through midsummer. This plant was known in the Middle Ages and greatly valued for its medicinal properties. In Germany comfrey is known as *Beinwurz*, which means 'leg-root', and it was given this name because it is extremely useful for treating diseased and injured bones. Both the leaves and the roots of the comfrey are still greatly prized.

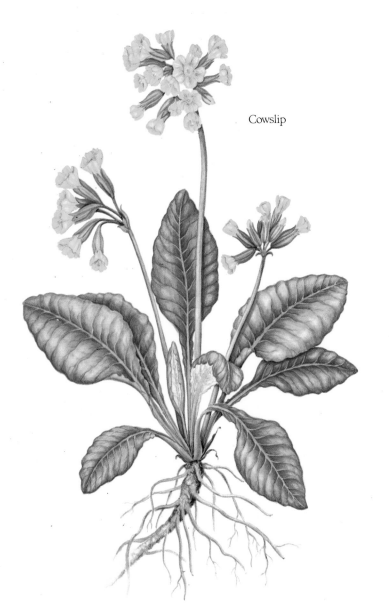

Cowslip

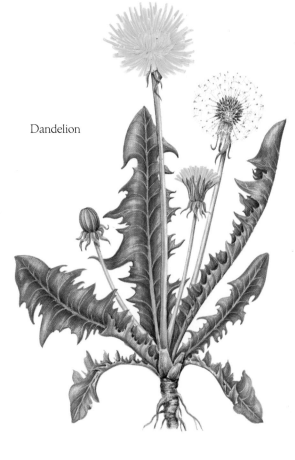

Dandelion

Cowslip

Primula officinalis

Violets, coltsfoot and the yellow flowers of the cowslip are among the first harbingers of spring, announcing the awakening of nature and bringing expectation of sunshine and balmy days to come. In the past the meadows in the countryside used to be full of a riot of gorgeous yellow cowslips in the spring, but our modern artificial fertilizers have all but wiped them out there now. However, cowslips, commonly known as marsh marigolds, can still survive in open lowland woods and forests, in ditches, along the banks of streams and under fruit trees.* The cowslip has a hardy rootstock, and it doesn't lose its rosette of green leaves in the winter. The entire floral umbel has medicinal properties. The Swiss herbalist Father Kuenzle is particularly fond of cowslips. "All the different varieties of cowslip have healing properties", he says, "no matter whether they grow in meadows and woods or in the hills, no matter whether they are pale in color or deep yellow. Even so, the dark-yellow, powerfully fragrant varieties are definitely more potent than the others".

* Overpicking is one of the reasons for the scarcity of cowslip, so please respect any plants you find growing in the wild, and bear the conservation code in mind.

Dandelion

Taraxacum officinale

The dandelion is a member of the aster family and is common in meadows and along the sides of country paths: a field full of countless dandelions in blossom is a joy to behold. A tubular stem, up to around 8 in (20cm) high and containing a kind of milky sap, grows out of a rosette of jaggedly toothed leaves. In time the bright yellow blossoms at the tops of the stems produce the characteristic dandelion clocks — the sphere of feathery white seeds that are carried hither and thither by the wind.

Dandelion roots dug up in the spring are more potent than those dug up in the autumn. The juice of the entire dandelion plant has blood-purifying properties and forms the basis of an excellent course of treatment for cleaning out the system in the spring. The famous medieval herbalist J.T. Müller, also known as Tabernaemontanus, referred to the dandelion as a "blesseyed medickamente", and he claimed that the juice of the roots and the stems had a miraculous effect on disorders of the eyes, making the eyesight clear again and eliminating unpleasant flecks and specks.

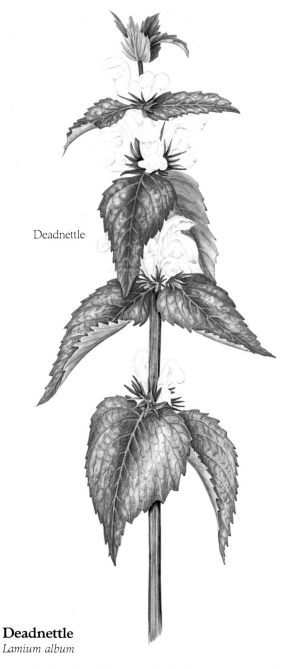

Deadnettle

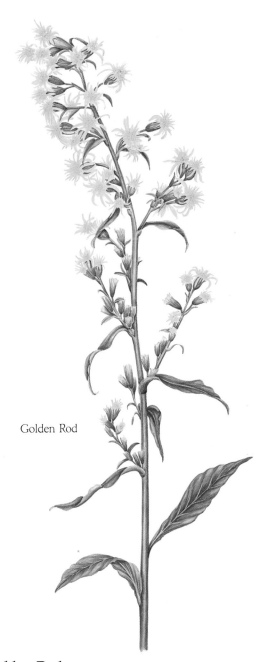

Golden Rod

Deadnettle
Lamium album

The white deadnettle belongs to the family of labiates (which includes mint, thyme and rosemary), and grows in the same places as the ordinary stinging nettle. The leaves and overall appearance of the deadnettle are similar to those of the stinging nettle, but the former has a softer, gentler shape. The plant reaches heights of between 8 and 12 in (20 and 30cm) and the creamy-white flowers grow in whorls around the stalks, nestling above the leaves. The flowers have a delicate, honey-like fragrance. The deadnettle blooms on slopes, railway embankments, along the edges of meadows and fields, in hedgerows and along fences and country paths.

The yellow deadnettle, or yellow archangel (*Lamium galeobdolon*), is distinguished from the white deadnettle only by its yellow flowers; it has the same whorled flower and leaf arrangement. The yellow archangel prefers open lowland forests, low ground and embankments and shady spots, in contrast to the white deadnettle, which loves the sunshine.

The leaves and flowers of both varieties have medicinal properties, and they have roughly the same potency. In the Middle Ages the white blossoms were used as a hair dye, producing a yellowish tint.

Golden Rod
Solidago virgo aurea

Golden rod is most commonly found at the edges of woods and forests in mountainous regions, in man-made forest clearings, and on meadowy slopes. The bushy stem reaches a height of about 2 ft 6 in (80cm) and bears golden-yellow sprays of flowers. Both the blooms and the leaves have a cooling effect and the plant itself is surrounded by a tangibly soothing aura. Simply seeing golden rod growing in the countryside is calming in itself, and country folk say that there is a gentle and helpful angel standing next to each plant. Golden rod blossoms in late summer; the fragrance of the blossoms is balmy and mild, contrasting sharply with that of the naturalized Canadian golden rod (*Solidago canadiensis*), which is much taller and grows in dense profusion at the edges of woods, in clearings and along the shores of lakes. Whereas ordinary golden rod is similar to the smaller mullein, the Canadian golden rod has fan-like panicles of yellow flowers, which are pointed at the ends.

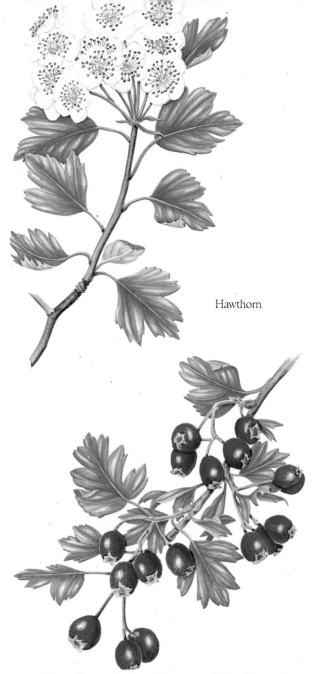

Hawthorn

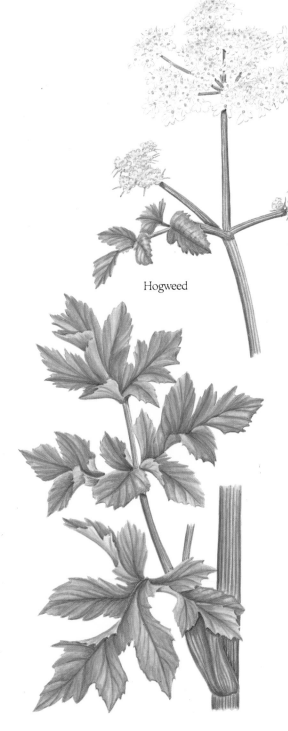

Hogweed

Hawthorn (May, Maytree, Mayflower)

Crataegus monogyna

The hawthorn is a medium-sized thorny shrub which can grow into a tree, reaching heights of up to 20ft (7m) or more. The leaves have from three to five lobes and are shiny on both sides. The white blossoms appear in abundant umbels and have a distinctive scent; the fruits are bright red and have a mealy consistency. The hawthorn grows in thickets and underbrush, in both evergreen and deciduous and forests, and along the edges of fences and hedgerows. There is an old legend that says the first hawthorn bush grew from the staff of St. Joseph. The lovely star-shaped blossoms appear in the spring, the bright red, barrel-shaped fruits in the autumn.

Hogweed (Cow Parsnip)

Heracleum sphondylium

This umbelliferous plant grows to a height of between 2 and 4 ft (60-120cm). It has ribbed, hollow stems and lobed leaves that are shaped rather like an animal's paw and that are covered with very coarse hairs. It can be found everywhere in the countryside: in meadows and pastures, along embankments and field boundaries, at the edges of woods and forests, on the banks of rivers, and in open deciduous and pine forests where there is not too much undergrowth. The umbels are large and flat, and they sometimes curve downwards at the edges. The color of the blossoms ranges from yellowish-white to greenish-yellow to a very light pink. You can't miss the cow parsnip in meadows and at the edges of fields, as it is usually taller than all the other plants around it. The hollow stems smell and taste rather like carrots, and in the spring they can be diced and used as a tasty addition to salads, together with the young leaves and shoots. Caution: Cow parsnip closely resembles water hemlock, which is a poisonous plant found in similar environments.

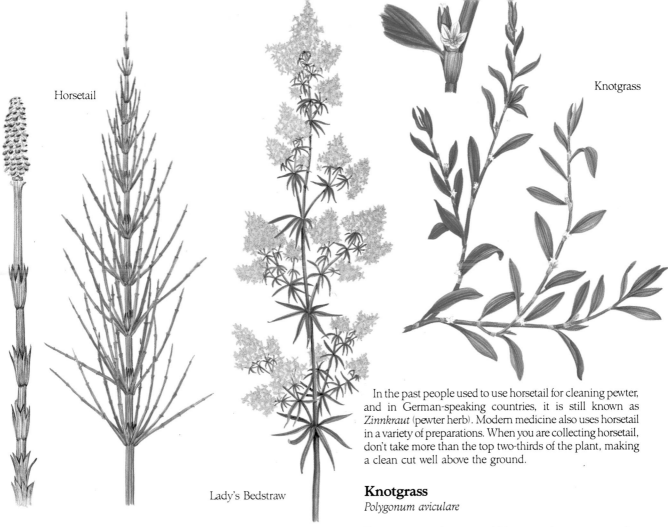

Horsetail

Knotgrass

Lady's Bedstraw

In the past people used to use horsetail for cleaning pewter, and in German-speaking countries, it is still known as *Zinnkraut* (pewter herb). Modern medicine also uses horsetail in a variety of preparations. When you are collecting horsetail, don't take more than the top two-thirds of the plant, making a clean cut well above the ground.

Knotgrass
Polygonum aviculare

Knotgrass grows between cobblestones, along country paths, on wasteland, in cemeteries and everywhere else where the soil is not particularly fertile. It usually grows along the surface of the ground, and has thin, branching stems bearing tiny, stemless leaves with minuscule whitish-pink flowers at their bases.

Lady's Bedstraw
Galium verum

Lady's Bedstraw grows in hedgerows, along fences, at the edges of woods and forests, in meadows, on slopes and along field boundaries. There are three varieties of bedstraw: *Galium aparine*, which blooms the whole summer long and grows in fields, woodlands and next to fences; *Galium verum*, which has very fragrant golden-yellow blossoms; *Galium molugo*, or hedge bedstraw, which has delicate, yellowish-white blossoms that look similar to those of maiden's breath (or gypsophila), but they are more compact, and they have a pungent, honey-like fragrance.

Lady's bedstraw has more potent medicinal properties than the white-flowered hedge bedstraw, but both of them are wonderful medicinal plants. The upright flower-bearing stems which grow out of the rootstock have delicate green leaves, and the plant bears these leaves the whole year round, even through the winter in areas where it doesn't snow. The leaves are similar to woodruff leaves, but there is no danger of confusing the two, as bedstraw leaves are much larger.

Midwives used to lay out the beds of women in childbirth with fresh lady's bedstraw, and it is claimed that this made the delivery easier.

Horsetail
Equisetum arvense

Horsetail grows in damp, sandy soil in fields, along the edges of woods and the banks of streams, and on meadowy slopes and railway embankments, but it likes loamy soil best of all. There are a number of different varieties of horsetail, all of which are non-flowering plants which reproduce through spores. In the spring the scaly, yellowish-brown spore-bearing stems of the horsetail appear. They reach lengths of 6 to 8 in 15-20cm and look rather like thin pencils. Once the wind has distributed the spores, these fruit-stems disappear again, and it is only then that the green haulms of the horsetail start to grow. By mid-spring a sterile leafless stalk appears, reaching a length of up to 2 ft (60cm) and producing small, regularly-spaced shoots. With the shoots these stalks resemble either little Christmas trees or horses' tails (hence the name), depending on your point of view. Horsetail has very deep roots through which it obtains a great deal of nourishment from the ground, making it a highly undesirable weed on arable land.

Only the infertile summer fronds of the horsetail have medicinal properties, not the spore-bearing stems. Strangely enough, horses and cattle get sick if they eat this plant. One variety of horsetail — the great horsetail — is poisonous, and shouldn't be taken internally under any circumstances, but it can be used for making infusions for medicinal baths. It is much taller than the common horsetail and has stalks as thick as an adult's finger. It grows in damp, swampy meadows and alpine pastures.

25

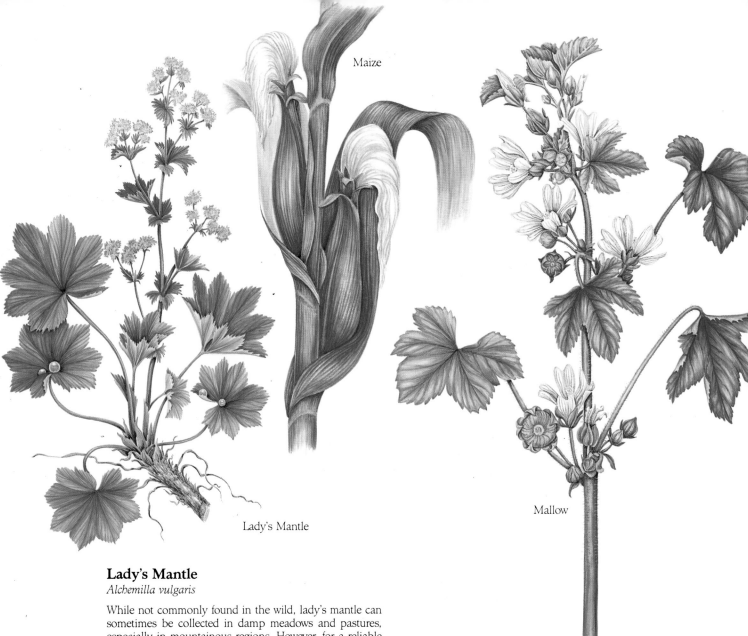

Maize

Lady's Mantle

Mallow

Lady's Mantle
Alchemilla vulgaris

While not commonly found in the wild, lady's mantle can sometimes be collected in damp meadows and pastures, especially in mountainous regions. However, for a reliable source it is best cultivated in the garden. The leaves are kidney-shaped, with either five or nine lobes. The small, greenish-yellow flowers are not particularly attractive. In the early morning large dewdrops collect in the leaves and in the sunlight they look like jewels resting in green bowls. Lady's mantle is a hardy plant — it doesn't lose its green leaves in the winter and it blooms again in the spring. The whole of the flowering plant has medicinal properties. In antiquity lady's mantle was regarded as a holy plant.

It you want to have ruddy cheeks, then try drinking lady's mantle tea for a few days! Father Kuenzle, the well-known Swiss herbalist, sings this plant's praises. "Every pregnant woman should drink large quantities of lady's mantle tea in the last eight to ten days before giving birth", he says. "If this gift of Providence were more widely known, then there would be fewer widowers, and fewer children without mothers".

Maize
Zea mays

The feathery tassels that grow out of the ends of maize cobs have medicinal properties. They should be picked before the corn on the cobs turns yellow.

Mallow
Malva neglecta

Mallow usually grows near stables and compost heaps, along the edges of buildings and in unpaved open spaces. The fibrous roots have a sweetish taste. The stalk, which bends over slightly, reaches a length of 1 to 2 ft (30-60cm) and bears long-stemmed, roundish leaves. The small, trumpet-like, whitish-pink flowers grow out of the stalks and ripen into round green fruits that have a rather cheese-like consistency. The wild mallow (*Malva sylvestris*) reaches a height of around 6 ft (150cm); its grass-green leaves have between three and seven lobes, and the light-pink blossoms grow out of the leafstems in bunches. The wild mallow also has medicinal properties, but it cannot be compared with the ordinary mallow, which is more potent than all the other varieties of the *Malva* genus, which includes the hibiscus and the hollyhock. Mallow contains emollients that help to soften hardened tissues. The stems, leaves and flowers can be collected from early spring to early fall, and the roots are a good remedy for whooping cough.

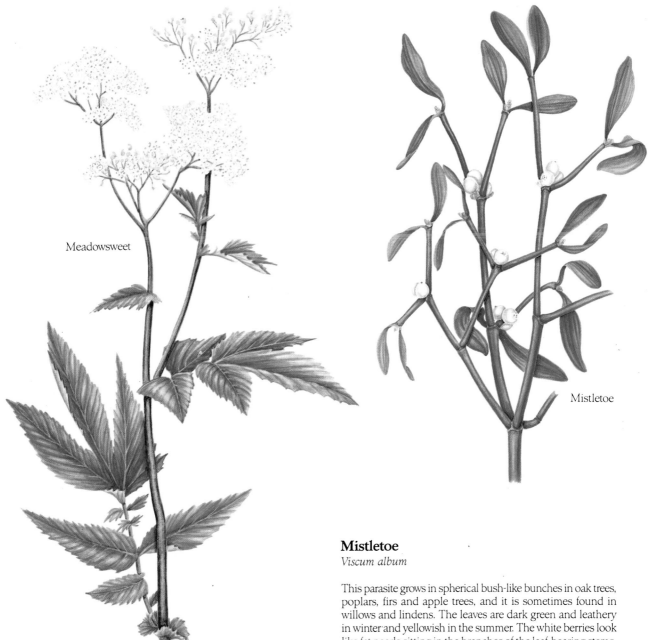

Meadowsweet

Mistletoe

Mistletoe
Viscum album

This parasite grows in spherical bush-like bunches in oak trees, poplars, firs and apple trees, and it is sometimes found in willows and lindens. The leaves are dark green and leathery in winter and yellowish in the summer. The white berries look like fat pearls sitting in the branches of the leaf-bearing stems. The juice of the poisonous berries is very sticky and viscous. The stickiness of the berries is the key to the mistletoe's propagation, for they adhere to the feathers of birds and are thus carried from tree to tree. Its medicinal properties coincide with the colder weather of late fall and early spring.

In the past, mistletoe was regarded as a magical plant, and in the pre-Christian era the priests and druids believed it to be a holy plant with mysterious and mystical healing properties that could cure any illness. And it really is a mysterious plant: it grows without earth, it is propagated without seeds and it remains green and flourishing even in the frost and snow. There is an old tradition that lightning never strikes a tree in which mistletoe is growing. The flowers appear in the autumn, and the berries develop some time later. Blackbirds and thrushes are especially partial to the berries, as are migratory birds that pass through in the depths of winter. Beware, though, the berries are poisonous to humans.

In recent years mistletoe has gained medical recognition as an ingredient in medicines used to retard the development of tumors in preventive cancer therapy.

Meadowsweet
Filipendula ulmaria

This plant grows in damp, swampy places, both in meadows and at the edges of woods and forests, and also on the banks of streams and in damp ditches, marshes and swamps. It also often grows among raspberry plants if the ground is damp enough. Meadowsweet reaches a height of some 7 ft (200cm) and flowers in mid-summer, although sometimes on into September. The blooms are a yellowish-white, and they have a sweet, almost intoxicating fragrance that is reminiscent of bitter almonds. The smell travels a long distance. Since the medicinal properties of both the flowers and the roots are more or less the same, most people prefer to use the flowers. Meadowsweet tea is a diuretic, and it is said to encourage sweating and to reduce fever.

27

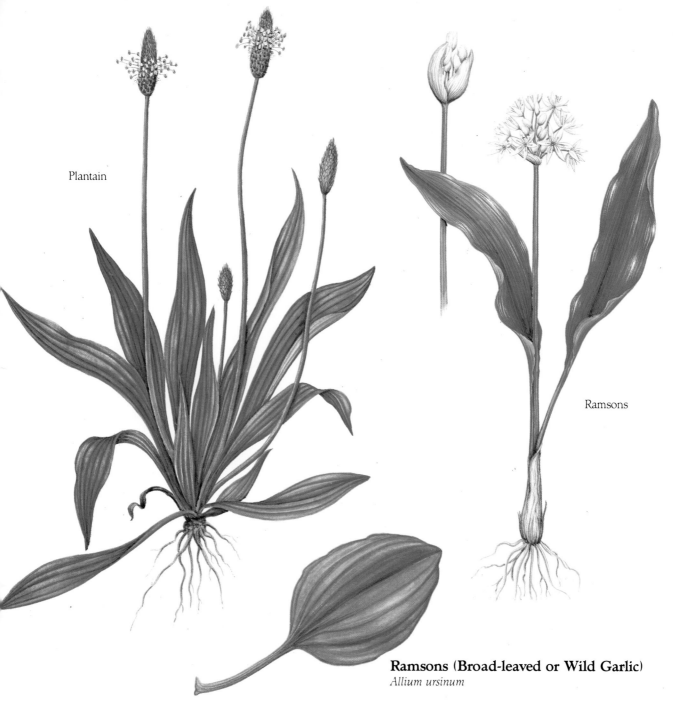

Plantain

Ramsons

Plantain
Plantago lanceolata

Both the plantain, buckhorn plantain and the great plantain (*Plantago major*), which belong to the same family, are common along the edges of fields and country paths and in meadows and pastures. In fact, it is difficult to find a country path anywhere that is not lined with great numbers of these plants. The leaves of both these varieties of plantain (which should be collected when the plants are in flower) have medicinal properties. The stem bearing the flowers rises up above the rosette of large leaves; the small white flowers of both varieties form a dense spike, but the spike of the great plantain is more rounded than that of the plantain. The leaves of the great plantain are broad, while those of the plantain are elongated and lance-like. Both varieties are hardy and keep their green leaves throughout mild winters.

Ramsons (Broad-leaved or Wild Garlic)
Allium ursinum

Ramsons is a shade-loving plant that grows in damp meadows, along the shady banks of streams and in undergrowth. It is often the first green plant to appear in the spring, covering the ground with a delightful light green carpet of leaves. Its leaves are similar to those of the lily of the valley and the common autumn crocus, both of which are poisonous. The leaves of the autumn crocus appear in the spring and it doesn't blossom until autumn, but even without these differences the pungent smell of garlic makes ramsons completely unmistakable. Although the leaves appear early, the pretty, long-stemmed white umbel doesn't sprout from the bulb until the middle of spring.

Ramsons is a very potent medicinal plant. According to an old folk tradition, after their winter hibernation bears purify their blood and their digestive systems by eating ramsons (hence its other name). Common garlic has similar blood-purifying properties, but ramsons is milder and even more potent.

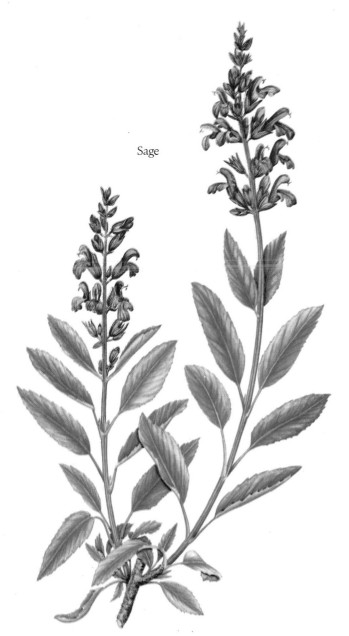

Sage

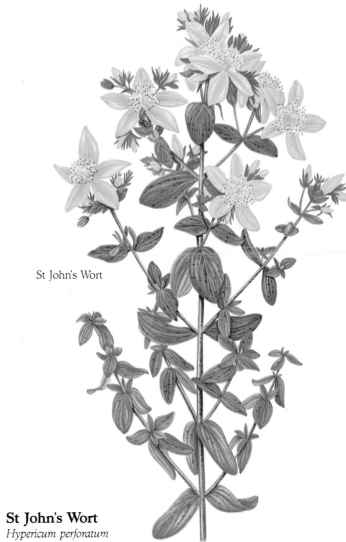

St John's Wort

St John's Wort
Hypericum perforatum

St John's wort can be found on dry embankments, in overgrown fields, at the edges of woods, in forest clearings, in abandoned gravel pits and on fallow land. The upright plant stem reaches a height of between 2 ft and 2 ft 4 in (60-70cm). The leaves are small and stemless, and the golden-yellow floral umbels appear at the end of shoots branching off the main stem. The flowers appear near to the time of the summer solstice, when the heat of the sun is at its most powerful.

The plant gives the impression of being literally drenched in light. If you hold the leaves and the flower petals up against the light, you will see a large number of translucent points, like pinpricks. This translucence is caused, by oil secreting cells. In Germany this plant is also called St John's blood because these oil glands make it look as though the blossoms and buds are speckled with tiny drops of blood. The flowers contain a reddish pigment, although this isn't immediately apparent, but if you rub the petals between your fingers, your skin will be covered with red juice. The entire plant (flowers, stalks and leaves) has medicinal properties, but only the blossoms and the buds are used for making St John's wort oil.

St John's wort has always been highly prized. For instance, Paracelsus was very impressed with its medicinal properties, speaking of it with great respect and saying that it was a plant in which God had hidden a great and wonderful secret. He claimed that simply being in the proximity of a flowering St John's wort plant was enough to help promote healing, and he advised his patients to place some under their nightcaps and beneath their pillows at night and to keep a bunch in their hands or place it in a little bag and wear it like a necklace.

Sage
Salvia officinalis

This medicinal plant should be grown in the home garden, since it is not often found in the wild. Its original home is the stony soil of coastal Yugoslavia and Herzegovina. Sage can grow into quite a large shrub. It has many branches, bearing furry, oval leaves with a silverish tinge and slightly toothed edges. Sage has a strong, pleasantly pungent and soothing aroma. It blooms in early to mid-summer and the color of the flowers ranges all the way from light to dark violet. The leaves can be picked and used for medicinal purposes throughout the summer and well into the autumn, and one should also remember the value of sage as a culinary herb! In antiquity sage was seen as a holy plant, and it was said that taking it regularly was a sure way of reaching a ripe old age.

In the summer the delightful blue flowers of the familiar meadow sage that grows on embankments and slopes are always a lovely, heart warming sight, but unfortunately the medicinal properties of this variety are negligible compared with those of garden sage. The only medicinal use for meadow sage is in the form of sage vinegar, which is an excellent embrocation for the bedridden to prevent bedsores.

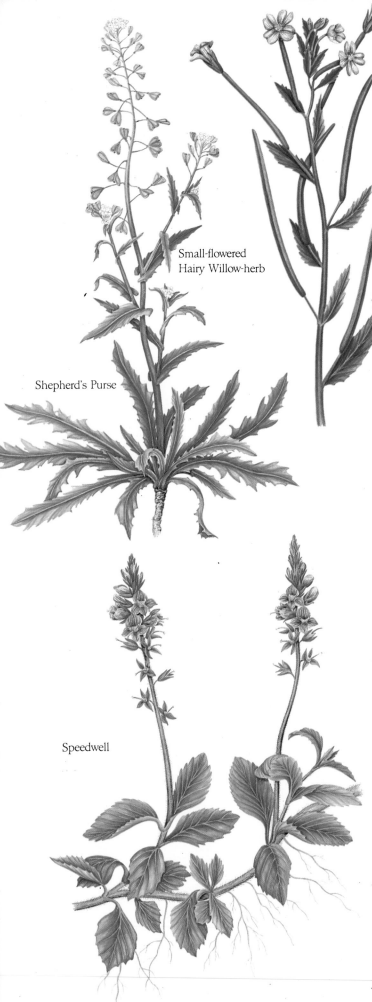

Small-flowered
Hairy Willow-herb

Shepherd's Purse

Speedwell

Shepherd's Purse
Capsella bursa pastoris

Shepherd's purse is a light green cruciferous plant that grows in beet and potato fields, along country paths, on fallow land, on fresh landfills and between rocks and stones. Lying flat on the ground directly above the upper end of the long tap-root is a rosette of leaves similar to that of the dandelion. The main stem reaches a height of between 8 and 16 in (20-40cm) and from it little heart-shaped bursicles (the "purses"), grow all the way up to the small white blossoms at the stem tips. Chickens and other domestic fowl are particularly fond of these bursicles. The entire plant has medicinal properties and should be picked in the spring. Shepherd's purse dies down in the summer heat, but shoots up again in the autumn. However in autumn the plant is very susceptible to a fungus infection, and you should try to avoid these infected plants when collecting your winter supply for drying. If the color does not remain an even green when the plants are dried this means that they are infected, and you should throw them away.

Shepherd's purse is a hardy plant, becoming completely dormant only in very frosty weather. It grows all over the world, and even in antiquity it was already known and valued for its ability to staunch bleeding. The same is true today: shepherd's purse is one of the best astringent agents (substances that stop bleeding) known to man, and it is an excellent remedy for all types of bleeding and hemorrhages.

Small-flowered Willow-herb
Epilobium parviflorum

There are several varieties of small-flowered willow-herb that have medicinal properties. With their delicate pointed leaves and their small, inconspicuous flowers, which can range from white to deep pink, they are clearly set off from the great hairy willow-herb, that has much larger flowers. The blossoms grow at the ends of longish green ovaries that contain large numbers of seeds encased in white, cotton-like fibres. Among the varieties of small-flowered willow-herb are the spear-leaved willow-herb, the small-flowered willow-herb, the broad-leaved willow-herb, the marsh willow-herb, the chickweed willow-herb, the square-stemmed willow-herbs and the alpine willow-herb. Although all of these varieties are small-flowered willow-herbs, the branching stems of some of the plants can sometimes reach heights of almost 2 ft 6in (80cm). The leaves and blossoms and also the stems (so long as they have not become woody) all have medicinal properties, and they can be collected in the spring.

The great hairy willow-herb is much larger than these smaller varieties; more of a shrub than a herb. Its flowers can be up to ten times bigger than those of the small-flowered willow-herb, and it has no medicinal properties. It can reach heights of between 5 ft and 5 ft 6 in (160 and 170cm), and its luminous, reddish-violet flowers can be seen from far away on the edges of woods and forests and in clearings. If they are picked in the early spring the leaves of this plant make a tasty addition to salads.

Speedwell
Veronica officinalis

Speedwell likes dry ground. It is widespread in meadows, pastures and clearings, on slopes and along the edges of paths and woods.

The stem reaches a height of around 1 ft (30cm). The leaves

have a silvery, whitish tinge to them, the floral ear is light blue, similar to forget-me-nots. Speedwell is a creeping plant that tends to stay close to the ground. The entire plant (stems, leaves and flowers) has medicinal properties, and is picked from early spring to mid-summer. The most potent variety, especially when it is growing beneath oak trees, is the so-called drug speedwell. Genuine speedwell doesn't lose its green leaves in the winter.

Stinging Nettle
Urtica urens

The stinging nettle grows along walls and paths, in hedgerows, fences, in thick underbrush, on wasteland and among rubble. It blossoms from mid- to late summer. Stinging nettles grow in particular abundance in places where the natural electromagnetic fields of the earth are unusually strong. There are two main types of stinging nettle — the larger stinging nettle (*Urtica dioica*) and the smaller common-or-garden nettle (*Urtica urens*). Both varieties have medicinal properties, but the sting of the garden nettle is stronger. Tall, four-sided stems bearing toothed, bristly leaves grow from a many-branched yellowish rootstock. The stem is full of long, tough fibres that were at one time used for making a kind of coarse cloth, similar to linen. The leaves, stalks, blossoms and roots all have medicinal properties. However, the roots lose these properties as soon as the nettle blooms, so they must be dug up before this happens.

The larger stinging nettle reaches a height of between 3 and 6 ft (100-150cm), while the smaller garden nettle grows up to about 16 in (40cm). The larger variety has either male or female flowers, which are wind pollinated. The smaller garden nettle (*Urtica urens*) has both male and female blossoms on the same plant and has no rootstock. The stinging nettle is one of those plants with which we all become acquainted at a very early age — it makes its presence stingingly felt when we come into contact with it! It grows all over the world, except in southern Africa and the polar regions.

Thyme
Thymus serpyllum

Thyme is another member of the labiate family. It grows along the boundaries between fields, on sunny meadows and slopes, on the edges of woods and forests, between stones, and near anthills. Thyme needs sunshine and warmth, and it grows close to the ground to make the most of the warmth radiated by the earth. The woody stems lie horizontally on the ground and shoots reaching heights of about 1 ft (30cm) grow up vertically from these stems. The leaves are small and oval, and the fragrant flowers are even smaller than the leaves, ranging in color from light to dark violet. Thyme blooms between early and late summer, and has an attractive, spicy fragrance. The plant usually grows in the form of dense bushes. These cushions are very popular with bumblebees, honeybees and other insects — a delightful sight in the summer. Every part of the plant has medicinal properties.

This wonderfully fragrant plant is one of my own personal favorites. In some parts of Europe it is considered a holy plant, dedicated to the Virgin Mary, and in Austria wreaths and garlands of thyme are still taken to church to be blessed on the festival of Corpus Christi. Thyme is a herb that can be used in an unusually wide variety of ways, both in the kitchen and in the treatment of illnesses. It has been in use as a medicinal plant since the Middle Ages.

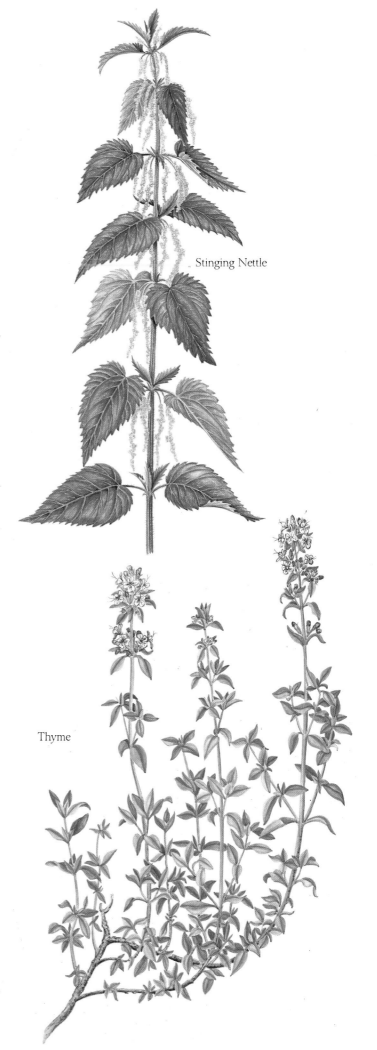

Stinging Nettle

Thyme

31

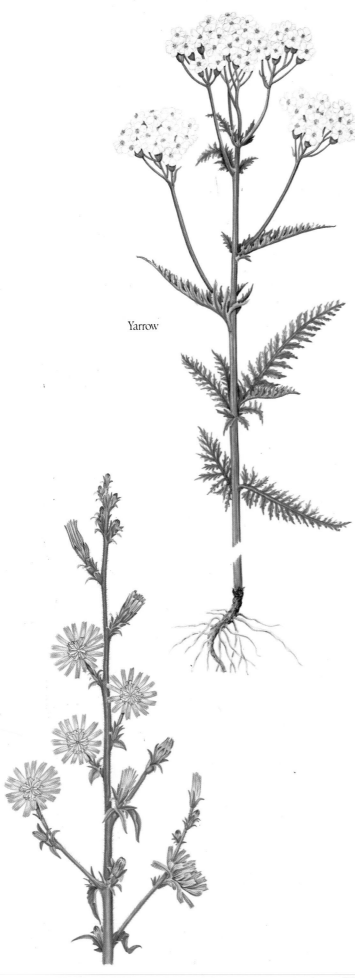

Yarrow

Yarrow
Achillea millefolium

Yarrow grows along the edges of country paths and field boundaries and on meadows, hills, slopes, embankments and mountainsides. The plants reach a height of 12 to 16 in (30-40cm). The yarrow blooms from early summer until frost, and the color of its flowers ranges from white to reddish. Yarrow has a very important place in traditional folk medicine, and in some European countries it is known as a cure all for it can be of help in the treatment of almost all known illnesses and complaints. It is one of the oldest medicinal plants known to man, and doctors all through the ages have always valued it very highly. It is said that yarrow regulates the "bodily juices", and it certainly does stimulate the production of fresh blood cells in the bone marrow, which may well be the reason for its unusually wide range of medical uses. In Austria yarrow is known as *Bauchwehkräutl* or bellyache herb because of its value in the treatment of diarrhea and dysentery. Both the blossoms and the leaves have medicinal qualities. The leaves should be collected in the spring. They have a pleasant flavor and, apart from being used as a medicine, they can also be chopped up finely and used as a garnish for salads and other dishes.

Wild Chicory (Succory)
Cichorium intybus

Wild chicory grows along country paths and field boundaries, in hedgerows and fallow fields, and anywhere else where it can find good-quality loamy soil. From a rosette of coarsely-toothed leaves at the base grows a tall, stiff and rather bare stem, with small, coarse-haired leaves and large, bright-blue flowers like shining stars at the ends of the bare shoots. The flowers of this plant were among my favorite flowers when I was a child, and whenever I see them now I am always reminded of many magical childhood experiences. The luminous blue flowers exercised a magnetic attraction on me, and when I touched them and stroked them I often had the feeling that they were the home of a host of benevolent angels who were particularly fond of small children.

There is a delightful old Silesian story about the origin of the wild chicory plant. It is said that, in the days when Our Lord was still on this earth in human form, he stopped during one of his journeys and asked a hard-hearted young lady for a little refreshment. The girl was waiting for her sweetheart, however, and she couldn't be bothered to help the stranger. She brushed him off brusquely and, when her sweetheart finally arrived some time later, the young man couldn't find her anywhere. Instead, a tall, hard-stemmed plant stood there by the wayside, and its beautiful flowers seemed to be gazing at him sadly, as if they were big blue eyes. The story goes that the proud maiden must now wait by the wayside until Our Lord finally returns. It is also said that this was the fate of many hard-hearted people, and in Germanic folklore wild chicory is therefore called *Armersünderblume* (poor sinners flower). The flowers of wild chicory open only when the sun is shining.

2. Prevention is Better than a Cure

We are all well aware of the fact that prevention really is better than a cure, but very few of us actually take the trouble to do anything about it. Most people seem to take good health for granted, and they don't seem capable of understanding that it is really a gift of providence and one of the most precious possessions we have. On the contrary, making lots of money and climbing the social and professional ladders are usually regarded as being much more important in our modern world than health. The simple fact that we need a healthy body if we are going to achieve all these worldly aims is something that people realize only when they become seriously ill and are forced to change their ways whether they want to or not. But we really don't have to wait until it's too late — with a healthy lifestyle and good preventive treatment with medicinal herbs, we need not get sick in the first place.

The medicinal herbs in God's garden are a wonderful gift, and it pays to make use of them. Unlike synthetic, chemical products, the healing properties of herbs are universal — they don't simply help to cure diseases, they also help to strengthen our bodies' resistance, protecting us from all sorts of illnesses that we might otherwise be subject to.

No car owner would dream of waiting until his car actually breaks down before taking it in to have it serviced, and our bodies need at least as much care and attention as our cars. This chapter contains a selection of recipes that will help you give your body a thorough cleaning-out and service, and if you follow the advice given here, you will be able to avoid many unnecessary repairs; procedures that are much more time-consuming and troublesome than a timely bit of prevention would have been.

If you are a little suspicious of herbal medicine in general these recipes provide a good way to gain confidence in it. Once you have experienced the invigoration and relief that one feels after taking a treatment course (the spring is the best time for this), you will develop a much more natural and relaxed attitude to medicinal herbs, for you will have first-hand knowledge of their value.

Where you came across an asterisk (*), refer to the relevant recipe in Chapter 5.

Dandelion Stems

The dandelion is at its most potent in the spring when it's in flower, and it's a good idea to take advantage of this fact and give your body a two-week treatment with fresh dandelion stalks. Eat ten raw, freshly-picked dandelion stems every day for the whole two weeks, washing them carefully beforehand and chewing them very thoroughly. Don't cut off the flowers before washing the plants. If you've been feeling tired and listless this treatment will perk you up very quickly.

Horsetail Tea

I would advise anyone over forty to drink one cup of horsetail tea* everyday. It helps to stop the onset of gout, rheumatism and the other similar complaints that tend to appear as one gets older. Make each cup of tea last a whole day, taking little sips at regular intervals.

Mistletoe Tea

The mistletoe is a very important medicinal plant; it helps to regulate the blood pressure and tones up the entire circulatory system. I would advise anyone who wants to do their body a favor to treat themselves to a six-week course of mistletoe tea* once every year. Drink three cups of tea every day for the first three weeks, two cups a day for the next two weeks and then one cup a day in the final week. By the end of the six weeks you'll find that your blood pressure has returned to normal, no matter whether it was too high or too low.

If you want to keep your circulatory system toned up and your blood pressure normal, drink one cup of mistletoe tea every day of the year.

N.B. Mistletoe berries are poisonous.

Nettle Tea

You do the common stinging nettle a great disservice when you call it a weed, for it is really one of the most important medicinal plants. It has blood-purifying properties and also helps to stimulate the production of fresh blood cells, all of which makes it an excellent choice if you want to give your body a thorough wash and brush-up.

Collect the young nettle shoots in the early spring and take three cups of nettle tea every day for four weeks. Drink one cup of tea in the early morning before breakfast and two more cups during the course of the day. It's important to drink the tea very slowly, one little sip at a time.

You can repeat this treatment again in the autumn if you want, when the second batch of shoots appear. It's a good idea to collect and dry a good supply of nettles in the spring and autumn so that you have enough for one cup of nettle tea every day of the year, as this will strengthen your body's resistance to illnesses of all kinds.

Plantain Syrup

A syrup made from fresh plantain leaves helps to purify the blood and should be taken before every meal. Adults should take a tablespoonful, children a teaspoonful.

There are two basic ways of making plantain syrup:

1. Mince four generous handfuls of freshly-washed plantain leaves, and then add a little water to the minced leaves to make the mixture more fluid. Mix in 9 oz (250g) of honey and 11 oz (300g) of unrefined cane sugar, and then heat the mixture up gently, stirring it constantly, and removing it from the heat just before it comes to the boil. Once the mixture has cooled you can pour it into some clean jam jars and store it in the refrigerator.

2. Take a large ceramic or glass container and fill it with alternating layers of freshly-picked and washed plantain leaves, and unrefined cane sugar. Give the layers a little time to steep and settle, and then add more layers of plantain leaves and sugar until the container is completely full again. Then seal the mouth with several layers of plastic film, making sure that the seal is completely airtight, and bury the container in a protected spot in the garden. (Take care to cover the mouth of the jar with a piece of wood before you shovel in the earth, otherwise you may make a hole in the plastic film!) The steady, gentle heat from the soil will make the sugar and plantain mixture start to ferment. Dig the container up after eight weeks and transfer the syrup into a big cooking pot. Place the pot on the stove and bring the syrup to the boil, very slowly and gently. Remove it from the heat as soon as it boils and allow it to cool before transferring it into glass bottles.

Ramsons (Broad-leaved Garlic)

Ramsons is a good agent for purifying the blood and cleaning out the stomach and the digestive system. It's a good idea to give yourself a treatment with ramsons in the spring, when it is at its most potent. The green leaves should be collected in early spring, before the flowers appear, and eaten raw. If you wash the leaves and chop them up finely you can use them both as a flavoring and as a garnish for all sorts of savory dishes. Spinach tastes lovely if you cook it with a few leaves of ramsons, and they also make a tasty addition to fresh salads.

St John's Wort Tea

St John's wort is very valuable in the treatment of nervous and mental disorders. The onset of sexual maturity in puberty is usually a very trying and stressful time for young girls especially, and they often react with nervous irritation, disturbed sleep and irregular or troublesome periods. Taken in good time, St John's wort can help to alleviate these symptoms, and I often advise growing girls to drink two cups of St John's wort tea* every day as a preventive measure. Drink two cups in the course of the day, taking care to sip it slowly.

Yarrow Tea

The famous hydrotherapist and naturopath Father Sebastian Kneipp often used to say that women would spare themselves a great deal of trouble if only they would take a cup of yarrow tea every now and then. I couldn't agree more — every woman should know and take advantage of yarrow's wonderful healing properties. It can be of tremendous help in the treatment of complaints such as irregular periods and problems during the menopause. It's a good idea to drink a cup of yarrow tea every day the whole year round. Drink the tea slowly, one sip at a time.

Thyme Tea

In my experience, drinking a cup of thyme tea* in the mornings instead of black tea or coffee can really work wonders. Your stomach will be very grateful to you, and you'll find that you feel fresher and more wide-awake and full of get-up-and-go. If you have a tendency to start the day with slight coughing fits you'll also find that these will ease up.

Four Seasons Herbal Tea

Early spring is the time to go out into the countryside and to start collecting herbs. The first medicinal plant of the year is the coltsfoot, and the last is the rose, whose petals must be collected in the autumn. The herbs in this four seasons mixture are collected in the order in which they are listed below — which is more or less the order of their appearance. In autumn they can then be mixed together to make a really healthy herbal tea. Take one heaping teaspoonful of this herbal mixture for each cup of tea. Pour on hot water and let the herbs steep for half a minute before sieving them off. Take one cup every day with your evening meal and drink it slowly, one sip at a time.

The mixture is made of equal parts of the following:

Coltsfoot flowers (and leaves, later in the season)
Cowslips (take the entire flowerhead)
Violet leaves and flowers
Lungwort flowers
Common sorrel (also known as cuckoo sorrel) flowers
Ground ivy flowers (just a few of these, for flavor)
Stinging nettle shoots
Lady's mantle leaves and flowers
Speedwell leaves, flowers and stems
Strawberry leaves
Blackberry shoots
Raspberry shoots
Elderberry shoots (and flowers, later in the season)
Daisies
Lime leaves (picked while the sun is shining, if possible)
Chamomile (picked while the sun is shining)
Meadowsweet flowers
Calendula flowers
Woodruff leaves, flowers and stems
Thyme leaves, flowers and stems
Lemon balm leaves, flowers and stems
Peppermint leaves, flowers and stems
Yarrow (picked while the sun is shining, if possible; half a measure only)
Flowers of the smaller mullein (picked while the sun is shining, if possible)
St John's wort flowers (picked while the sun is shining, if possible)
Marjoram leaves and flowers (wild marjoram)
Small-flowered willow-herb leaves, flowers and stems
Pine needles
Bedstraw leaves, flowers and stems
Rose petals (the color of the roses doesn't matter, but only the petals from organically fertilized plants should be used)

Springtime Tea

The following herbal tea mixture is excellent for purifying the blood. It's advisable to drink two cups of this tea every day for as long as the fresh herbs are available.

To make the mixture take ½ oz (15g) of nettle leaves, 1½ oz (50g) of fresh young elderberry buds, ½ oz (15g) of dandelion root and 1½ oz (50g) of cowslips and mix them well.

Use one heaped teaspoonful of this mixture for each cup of tea. Pour on hot water and let the herbs steep for half a minute before sieving them off. Drink two cups of this tea in the course of the day, taking care to sip it slowly. If you have a sweet tooth you can add a little honey.

Autumn Tea

In autumn, when the onset of wet, cold weather heralds the beginning of the flu season, it's a good idea to take some timely preventive measures. A tea made from the following herbal mixture provides good protection against flu.

Mix ½ oz (10g) of elderberry blossoms, ¼ oz (5g) of coltsfoot, ¼ oz (5g) of chamomile, ¼ oz (5g) of linden leaves, ½ oz (10g) of finely-chopped dandelion root, ¼ oz (5g) of wild strawberry leaves and ¾ oz (15g) of meadowsweet.

Use one heaping teaspoonful of this mixture for each cup of tea. Pour on hot water and let the herbs steep for five minutes (this is because of the dandelion roots) before straining them off. Drink three cups of this tea a day, taking care to sip it slowly. Divide the first cup into two equal portions, taking one of them before breakfast and the other one half an hour afterwards. Put the rest of the tea in a thermos and drink it in the course of the day. You may also take one teaspoonful of Swedish bitters* a day, dissolved in a little of the mixed herb tea described above.

Swedish Bitters

Swedish bitters* are an excellent preventive remedy for influenza and pains and illnesses of all kinds. Take one teaspoonful every morning and evening in a little water or herb tea.

This wonderful concoction is an indispensable aid to health that no household should be without. The recipe was invented by Dr. Samst, a Swedish physician whose entire family reached a ripe old age, thanks to the help of his Swedish bitters. For everyday use you can strain off some of the tincture into small bottles, which should be kept in a cool, dark place. The potency of Swedish bitters becomes greater the longer it is allowed to stand.

3. The Gentle Way to Health

Medicinal herbs have been growing in God's garden ever since the dawn of history. Unfortunately, we have now all but forgotten them and the blessings that they can bring. We have become restless and impatient, our scientific and technological successes have made us arrogant and lazy, and the continuous march of industrial progress is taking us further and further away from our roots in nature. The industrial revolution has changed us and our world in many ways, and not all of these changes have been for the better.

Stress, affluence and excess have created a whole series of new illnesses. For many people being ill has become a way of life, for it brings them the care, sympathy and attention that very few healthy people in our anonymous cities have much chance of getting. The doctor's waiting room is often more than just a waiting room — it has become a meeting place, providing a forum for the everyday social intercourse of country, village and even town life that we used to be able to take for granted. And in the course of all the other rapid changes that have taken place in this century, there has also been a radical change in people's attitudes to their own health.

Many people have completely lost any sense of proportion and moderation, especially when it comes to taking medicines. Even the most minor complaints are now often treated with massive doses of powerful antibiotics and chemicals. Nobody has the time to stop to think any more; the only thing that seems to matter is the achievement of rapid results. It's hardly surprising that more and more responsible doctors are now issuing dire warnings about the possible results of the addiction to prescribed drugs that is increasing all the time. If only people would make use of medicinal herbs a little more often, instead of rushing off to the doctor and the chemist's to get an easy solution in the form of a bottle of pills, they would find that this vicious circle can be broken, and one of my most heartfelt wishes would come true.

This chapter contains an alphatical list of the illnesses and complaints that you can treat with medicinal herbs from God's garden as with non-prescription drugs from the chemist's shop, but without any side-effects.

Where you come across an asterisk (*), refer to the relevant recipe in Chapter 5.

ABSCESSES

Calendula Ointment
Apply ointment* directly to the abscess.

Cow Parsnip Dressing
Wash some freshly-picked cow parsnip leaves and crush them to a pulp on a wooden chopping board using a rolling pin. Apply the fresh pulp directly to the abscess and cover it gently with a warm cloth. If you wish you may use whole, instead of crushed, leaves to make these dressings, but remember to wash them first.

Horsetail Compresses
Put two generous handfuls of horsetails in a sieve and heat them up over a pot of boiling water. When the horsetail is piping hot, wrap it up in a clean linen cloth and apply it directly to the affected area, binding it gently into place with another cloth. Leave this hot compress on for several hours, or put it on in the evening before you go to sleep and leave it on overnight.

Swedish Bitters
Apply a little undiluted Swedish bitters* to the abscess several times a day.

Home Remedy
Pour a little milk into a saucepan (just enough to cover the bottom completely) and add 4 oz (125g) of cottage cheese. Mix the milk and the cottage cheese well and then warm them up gently on a low heat, stirring constantly. When the mixture is warm (don't let it get too hot), spread it on a clean linen cloth and lay the cloth on your chest overnight, binding it into place with another cloth (and a layer of plastic film if you wish) to protect the bedclothes.

ACNE

Dandelion Root Tea
Drink half a cup of dandelion root tea* 30 minutes before breakfast and the other half 30 minutes after breakfast, taking care to sip it slowly.

Horseradish and Vinegar Mask

Put some freshly-grated horseradish in a glass bottle and pour in enough wine or fruit vinegar to cover it completely. Allow the mixture to stand in a warm place for ten days before using it. The mask should be applied twice a day — once in the morning and once in the evening. Moisten your face with cold water, apply the mask and leave it on for ten minutes. Then rinse it off, first with hot water and then with cold.

Nettle Tea

No other medicinal plant is better at purifying the blood and stimulating the production of fresh, healthy blood cells than the common stinging nettle. If you suffer from acne, avoid all rich, heavy foods and drink four cups of nettle tea* every day. Drink the tea slowly, one sip at a time.

Walnut Leaf Tea

Soak a heaped teaspoonful of finely chopped walnut leaves in a ½ pt (¼l) of water for twelve hours. Then heat the infusion up gently, strain off the walnuts leaves and add the liquid to the water you are going to use for washing your face.

AGE SPOTS (senile keratosis)

Bedstraw Ointment

Melt 1 lb (500g) of pure lard in a saucepan and add four generous handfuls of bedstraw. Proceed according to the standard recipe for ointment.*

Bedstraw Wash

These pigmented patches that appear on the

Some practical hints

Every illness usually has a whole series of different symptoms. For instance, if you have a bad cold you will probably have a runny nose, a cough and a hoarse throat, all at the same time. There's no need to make three separate herb teas to deal with these three symptoms; it's perfectly all right to mix equal quantities of the three different recipes to make one tea mixture. However, do remember not to drink the entire quantity at once: it's much more effective to spread the required amount over the day and to sip it slowly, instead of gulping it all down at once. The same principle applies when it comes to preventive remedies. In the flu season, for instance, it's a good idea to add a few drops of Swedish bitters to your tea.

There are no restrictions at all on mixing herbs to make your medicinal teas, even if the herbs you are using are for dealing with a wide variety of illnesses and symptoms. The medicinal herbs in God's garden know their way around the human body, and they always go to the place where they are needed. Nor do the different herbs compete with or neutralize one another if you take them together.

And another thing: don't be afraid that you might be overdosing. Your body won't have any trouble handling the quantities of tea suggested — after all, your kidneys actually need a minimum of four pints of liquid every day to be able to do their work properly! This does not mean, however, that you should go to the other extreme and start drinking huge quantities of herb tea. Medicinal herbs are most

effective when they are used in moderation, and adding a greater quantity of the herbs to your tea or bathwater will not make you get better any faster. It's much more important to tune yourself in to the healing powers of the herbs. Pay attention to your own body, listen to it and learn to open up to the gentle healing effects of the herbs, instead of allowing the illness to take control of you. Believe me, when it comes to getting well, your inner feelings are at least as important as choosing the right herbs and using them properly and in the right quantities.

Unless otherwise specified, the quantities mentioned in all the recipes refer to the dried herbs which you can buy from a herbal supplier. If you are willing to take the trouble to collect your own fresh herbs (which are more potent than dried ones) then you should replace each heaping teaspoonful of dried herbs with a handful of fresh ones. It doesn't matter if your hands are large, so that your handful is bigger than someone else's; the most important thing is to follow the instructions for preparing the tea precisely. Take particular care never to boil the herbs or to use water that is actually boiling, as this destroys all the active substances that they contain. And when you take a sitz bath or a full bath don't forget to get into bed and work up a sweat afterwards, as described in the individual recipes, as this is a very important part of the healing process. Where you come across an asterisk (*), refer to the relevant recipe in Chapter 5.

skin of elderly people can be treated effectively by bathing them with a bedstraw wash* every day.

Calendula Juice

To make the juice wash some fresh calendula stalks and run them through a juice extractor. Apply the juice to the affected areas several times a day.

Cedar Tincture

Apply cedar tincture* to the affected areas with cotton wool several times a day.

Houseleek Sap

Cut the houseleek leaves up lengthways and apply the sap directly to the pigment spots.

Swedish Bitters

Apply undiluted Swedish bitters* to the affected areas with cotton wool several times a day.

ALLERGIES (skin rashes)

Mallow Wash

Allergy rashes can be healed with the help of this mallow wash.

Soak two heaping teaspoons of mallow in 1 pt (½l) of cold water for twelve hours, then heat up the infusion gently and strain it. Bathe the affected area several times a day with the liquid.

Nettle Tea

Drink up to four cups of nettle tea* a day, taking care to sip it slowly.

ANXIETY

Hawthorn Tea

Drink two cups of hawthorn tea* during the day, taking care to sip it slowly.

Hawthorn Tincture

Take between four and ten drops of hawthorn tincture* a day.

Mistletoe Tea

Drink up to three cups of mistletoe tea* in the course of a day, taking care to sip it slowly.

APPETITE (Loss of)

Calamus Root Baths

It is important that your heart should be above the water level. Stay in the myrtle flag root bath* for twenty minutes, and don't dry yourself off when you get out; put on a dressing gown and get straight into bed, staying there for an hour so that you work up a good sweat.

Calamus Root Tea

Soak 1 level teaspoonful of myrtle flag root in ½ pt (¼l) of cold water (this makes enough for one cup) for twelve hours, and then heat up the infusion gently and strain it. Drink it slowly, taking small sips at regular intervals. Your appetite will soon return if you drink a cup of this tea each day and take one myrtle flag bath every week.

Hawthorn Tea

Drink two cups of hawthorn tea* in the course of the day, taking care to sip it slowly.

Hawthorn Tincture

Take between four and ten drops of hawthorn tincture* every day.

Sage Tea

Drink two cups of sage tea* in the course of the day, taking care to sip it slowly.

Swedish Bitters

Take three teaspoons of Swedish bitters* every day, dissolving each spoonful in half a cup of herb tea. Divide each of these three doses into two portions, taking one before eating and the other one afterwards.

Thyme Baths

It is important that your heart should be above the water level. Stay in the thyme bath* for twenty minutes, and don't dry yourself off when you get out; put on a robe and get straight into bed. Stay there for an hour so that you work up a good sweat.

Wild Chicory Tea

Drink one cup of wild chicory tea* in the morning, taking care to sip it slowly.

Yarrow Tea

Take two cups of yarrow tea* a day, drinking it as hot as you can bear it.

ATHLETE'S FOOT

Calendula Ointment

Apply calendula ointment to the affected areas

every day. Melt 1 lb (500g) of good quality lard in a saucepan and add four generous handfuls of finely-chopped calendula leaves, stalks and flowers. Proceed according to the standard recipe for ointment.

Calendula Wash
Pour 1 pt (½l) of hot water into a bowl containing a heaping tablespoonful of calendula leaves, stems and flowers and let the herbs steep for thirty seconds before straining them off and bathing your feet with the liquid.

BACK PAIN

Chestnut Compresses
Shell some fresh chestnuts and grind them up in a blender. Fill a pillowcase or cushion-cover loosely with the ground chestnuts and apply it to the affected area as a compress.

St John's Wort Oil
St John's wort oil* is of great value for the treatment for back pain. Gently massage it into the affected area.

Yarrow Tea
Take three to four cups of yarrow tea* a day, drinking it as hot as you can bear it and taking care to sip it slowly.

BARBER'S RASH

Horsetail Wash and Compresses
Barber's rash can be healed by bathing the affected areas several times a day with a horsetail wash.*

The drained horsetail left over from making the wash can be used in a hot compress. Wrap it in a clean cloth while it is still hot and apply it to the affected area. Leave the compress on until the herbs have cooled off, then reheat the wash and bathe the affected area with it.

BED-WETTING

Knotgrass Tea
Use one heaped teaspoonful of knotgrass for each cup of tea and soak it in the cold water for twelve hours. Then heat up the infusion gently and strain off the knotgrass. Drink four cups of this tea in the course of the day, taking care to sip it slowly.

It's a good idea to keep your day's supply in a pre-warmed thermos.

St John's Wort and Horsetail Tea
Mix equal parts of St John's wort and horsetail. Use one heaping teaspoonful of this mixture for each cup of tea. Pour on hot water and let the herbs steep for thirty seconds before straining them off. Drink one to two cups of the tea in the course of the day, taking care to sip it slowly. Eat solid foods only in the evening while you are using this treatment.

St John's Wort Sitz Baths
A St John's wort sitz bath* should be just deep enough to cover your kidneys. Stay in the bath for twenty minutes, and don't dry yourself off when you get out; put on a robe and get straight into bed. Stay there for an hour so that you work up a good sweat.

St John's Wort Tea
Drink two to three cups of St John's wort tea* in the course of the day, sipping it slowly.

Yarrow Sitz Baths
A yarrow sitz bath* should be just deep enough to cover your kidneys. Stay in the bath for twenty minutes, and don't dry yourself off when you get out; put on a robe and get straight into bed. Stay there for an hour so that you work up a good sweat.

BEE STINGS

See Insect bites.

BIRTHMARKS

Bedstraw Ointment
Bedstraw ointment is an excellent treatment for birthmarks.

Melt 1 lb (500g) of pure lard in a saucepan and add four generous handfuls of bedstraw. Proceed according to the standard recipe for ointment.*

Bedstraw Wash
Bathe the affected area with a bedstraw wash* every day.

Calendula Juice
Run some freshly-picked calendula stems through a juice extractor and apply the juice to the birthmark several times a day.

Cedar Tincture
Apply a little cedar tincture* to the birthmark several times a day with cotton wool.

Houseleek Sap
Take some fresh leek leaves, wash them, cut them into long thin strips and dab the sap which they exude on to the birthmark.

Swedish Bitters
Apply a little undiluted Swedish bitters* to the birthmark several times a day with a wad of cotton wool.

BLACKHEADS

Bedstraw Juice
Applied to the affected areas every day, freshly-pressed bedstraw juice brings about a rapid improvement. To make the juice take fresh bedstraw, wash it, and run it through a juice extractor without drying it off first. Apply the juice directly to the skin and let it dry.

Bedstraw Wash
Bathe your face with a bedstraw wash* every day.

BLADDER COMPLAINTS

Agrimony Tea
Drink three cups of agrimony tea* a day, taking care to sip it slowly.

Golden Rod Tea
Drink three to four cups of golden rod tea* a day, taking care to sip it slowly.

Plantain and Thyme Tea
Pour hot water into a cup containing a heaping teaspoonful of equal parts of plantain and thyme, and let the herbs steep for thirty seconds before straining them off. Drink the tea slowly, one sip at a time.

BLISTERS (on the feet)

Butterbur Leaves
Blisters on the feet can be both prevented and treated by putting freshly-picked butterbur leaves in your shoes.

Calendula Tea
Drink one or two cups of calendula tea* in the course of the day, taking care to sip it slowly.

Plantain Leaves
It's a good idea to put freshly-picked plantain leaves in your shoes when you go on walks and hikes, as they can prevent the formation of blisters. If you already have blisters, then putting these leaves in your shoes will help to dry them up.

BLOOD (purification of the)

Dandelion Roots
Fresh, raw dandelion roots also help to purify the blood. Wash the roots carefully under running water (use a brush) before eating them, and chew them very thoroughly.

Dried dandelion roots can be used to make tea. Take a heaping teaspoonful of dried dandelion root and soak it in a cupful of cold water for twelve hours. Then heat up the infusion gently, strain off the dandelion roots and divide the liquid into two equal portions. Take one portion half an hour before eating breakfast and the other one half an hour afterwards, and drink it slowly, one sip at a time. It's a good idea to put the tea in a pre-warmed thermos as soon as you make it, so that you don't need to heat it up again.

Deadnettle Tea
Drink one or two cups of deadnettle tea* a day, taking care to sip it slowly.

Herbal Mixture
Mix ½ oz (15g) of stinging nettle leaves, ½ oz (15g) of dandelion leaves, 1½ oz (50g) of elderberry buds and 1½ oz (50g) of cowslips. This mixture makes an excellent blood-purifying tea.

Use one heaped teaspoonful of the mixture for each cup of tea. Pour on hot water and let the herbs steep for thirty seconds before straining them off. Drink two cups of the tea in the course of the day, taking care to sip it slowly. If you have a sweet tooth you can add a little honey.

Meadowsweet Tincture
Fill a glass bottle with freshly-picked meadowsweet flowers and pour in enough 38-40% grain alcohol to cover them completely. Leave the sealed bottle to stand in a warm place for at least two weeks. Take between ten and fifteen drops of the tincture every day.

Nettle Tea

Drink up to four cups of nettle tea* a day, taking care to sip it slowly.

Ramsons (Broad-leaved Garlic)

Ramsons has excellent blood-purifying properties. The fresh leaves should be collected in the spring and eaten raw. Wash the leaves, chop them up finely, and sprinkle them on your food as you would fresh parsley. Spinach tastes lovely if you cook it with a few ramsons leaves, and they also make an excellent addition to salads.

Ramsons (Broad-leaved Garlic) Tincture

Drying ramsons destroys its potency, so the only way of benefiting from its wonderful healing properties all the year round is to prepare a supply of ramsons tincture.* Take between ten and fifteen drops of ramsons tincture four times a day, dissolving it in a little water.

Sage Tea

Drink one or two cups of sage tea* during the day, taking care to sip it slowly.

Speedwell and Nettle Tea

A mixture made of equal parts of speedwell and stinging nettles makes an excellent blood-purifying tea.

Use one heaped teaspoonful of the mixture for each cup of tea. Pour on hot water and let the herbs steep for thirty seconds before straining them off. Drink up to four cups of the tea a day, taking care to sip it slowly.

Swedish Bitters

Take three teaspoonfuls of Swedish bitters* a day, dissolving it in a little lukewarm water or one of the herb teas described here.

Walnut Leaf Tea

Drink one cup of walnut leaf tea* a day, taking care to sip it slowly.

Wild Chicory Tea

Drink one cup of wild chicory tea* in the early morning, taking care to sip it slowly.

Yarrow Tea

Drink one or two cups of yarrow tea* a day, taking care to sip it slowly.

BLOOD CELLS (stimulating the production of)

Celandine Tea

Drink two cups of celandine tea* a day, taking care to sip it slowly.

Nettle Tea

The common stinging nettle is a much underestimated plant. In addition to purifying the blood it also helps to stimulate the production of fresh blood cells. Drink up to four cups of nettle tea* a day, taking care to sip it slowly.

Wild Chicory Tea

Drink one cup of wild chicory tea* in the early morning, taking care to sip it slowly.

Yarrow Tea

Drink up to three cups of yarrow tea* in the course of the day, taking care to sip it slowly.

BLOOD-PRESSURE (high)

Club Moss Compresses

In some cases high blood-pressure can be caused by hyperactive kidneys. I used to have high blood-pressure myself, but I managed to get it back down to normal again by stuffing a small pillowcase with club moss and applying it to my kidneys as a compress.

Take a pillowcase or cushion cover and stuff it with 7 to 10 oz (200-300g) of dried club moss, depending on how large the compress needs to be. When you go to bed place the compress against kidneys and leave it there all night. This treatment is even more effective if you stuff the cushion with fresh club moss. You can also use this compress as a preventive measure, to keep your blood-pressure from going up in the first place.

Mistletoe Tea

Mistletoe is a truly amazing plant, which has the ability to balance the blood-pressure, bringing it back to normal, no matter whether it is too high or too low. Drink three cups of mistletoe tea* every day, taking care to sip it slowly.

Shepherd's Purse Tea

Shepherd's purse is another plant that helps to normalize both high and low blood-pressure. Drink two cups of shepherd's purse tea* every day, taking care to sip it slowly.

Home Remedy

Soak a small towel in cold water and then wring it out so that it is damp, but not dripping wet. Place the towel over your heart when you go to bed, covering it with a layer of plastic film to protect your clothes from the damp and a dry towel to keep the warmth in, and leave it on overnight.

Kneipp's "water treading" treatment is another excellent home remedy for high blood-pressure. Place a large bowl of cold water on the floor, step into it, then walk on the spot in the water. Begin with thirty steps (i.e., fifteen with each foot), working your way up slowly to sixty steps, and then reduce the number back down to thirty. You should take the same number of days to decrease the number of steps from sixty to thirty as you took to increase them from thirty to sixty. A similar effect can be achieved by walking barefoot on dew-covered grass in the early morning.

BLOOD-PRESSURE (low)

Mistletoe Tea

Drink three cups of mistletoe tea* every day, taking care to sip it slowly. It's a good idea to keep your day's supply in a pre-warmed thermos.

Shepherd's Purse Tea

Drink two cups of shepherd's purse tea* every day, taking care to sip it slowly.

BOILS

Bedstraw Juice

Wash some freshly-picked bedstraw, run it through a juice extractor and apply the fresh juice directly to the boil.

Bedstraw Tea

Let a cup of bedstraw tea* cool a little and then bathe the boil with it.

Cow Parsnip Dressings

Wash some freshly-picked cow parsnip leaves and crush them to a pulp on a wooden chopping board using a rolling pin. Apply the fresh pulp directly to the boil and bind it in place with a warm cloth. If you wish, you can make the dressings with whole leaves instead.

BREASTS (swollen)

Shepherd's Purse Compresses

Nursing mothers often suffer from swollen breasts. Hot shepherd's purse compresses are a good remedy for this complaint.

Put two generous handfuls of shepherd's purse in a large sieve and heat it up over boiling water. When the shepherd's purse is piping hot, wrap it in a clean linen cloth and apply it directly to the affected area, covering it with a thick towel to retain the heat.

BRONCHIAL CATARRH

Coltsfoot Juice

Coltsfoot juice can be made in the spring when the coltsfoot plants are ripe. Wash some freshly-picked coltsfoot leaves carefully and run them through a juice extractor. Take between two and three teaspoons of the freshly-made juice a day, dissolved in a cup of meat broth or a glass of warm milk.

Coltsfoot Syrup

Take a large ceramic or glass container and fill it with alternate layers of freshly-picked and washed coltsfoot leaves and unrefined cane sugar. Give it a little time to steep and settle, and then add more layers of coltsfoot leaves and sugar until the container is completely full again. Then seal the mouth with several layers of plastic film, making sure that the seal is completely airtight, and bury the container in a protected spot in the garden. (Cover the mouth of the jar with a piece of wood before you replace the earth, otherwise you may make a hole in the plastic film!) The steady, gentle heat from the soil will make the sugar and coltsfoot mixture ferment. Dig the container out again after eight weeks and transfer the syrup into a large cooking pot. Place the pot on the stove and gently bring the syrup to the boil. Remove it from the heat as soon as it boils, allow it to cool and then transfer it into glass bottles. Take one teaspoonful of this syrup every day, either neat or dissolved in a cup of herb tea.

Herbal Mixture

Mix equal parts of speedwell, coltsfoot leaves, lungwort and plantain. A tea brewed from this mixture is a good remedy for bronchial catarrh. Use one heaped teaspoonful of the mixture for each cup of tea. Pour on hot water and let the herbs steep for thirty seconds before straining them off. This tea is a little bitter, and if you wish you can sweeten it by dissolving a little honey or brown sugar in the hot water before pouring it over the herbs.

Plantain and Thyme Tea

Drink the tea as hot as possible, one sip at a time. Take four to five cups of plantain and thyme tea* a day, always making it just before you drink it.

Ramsons (Broad-leaved Garlic) Wine

This ramsons wine brings rapid relief from chest congestion.

Put a handful of ramsons flowers in a small saucepan, add ½ pt (¼l) of white wine, bring it to the boil briefly and then strain off the flowers. Make this quantity last the whole day long, taking little sips at regular intervals. If the wine is too bitter you can sweeten it with a little honey or syrup.

BRONCHITIS

Coltsfoot Tea

Use one heaping teaspoonful of a mixture made of equal parts of coltsfoot leaves and flowers for each cup of tea. Pour on hot water and let the herbs steep for thirty seconds before straining them off. Drink several cups of this tea in the course of the day, sipping it slowly, as hot as possible. You can sweeten the tea with honey if you wish.

Home Remedy

Pour a little milk into a saucepan (just enough to cover the bottom completely) and add 4 oz (125g) of cottage cheese. Mix the milk and the cottage cheese well and then warm them up gently on a low heat, stirring constantly. When the mixture is warm (don't let it become too hot) spread it on a clean linen cloth and lay the cloth on your chest overnight, binding it into place with another cloth and a layer of plastic film if you wish to protect the bedclothes.

Horsetail Tea

If you suffer from chronic bronchitis it's a good idea to drink horsetail tea regularly. Drink two to three cups of horsetail tea* every day, taking care to sip it slowly.

Plantain and Thyme Tea

Drink the tea as hot as possible, sipping it slowly. Take four to five cups of Plantain and thyme tea* a day, always making it just before you drink it.

BRUISES AND CONTUSIONS

Arnica Tincture

Apply a little arnica tincture* directly to the bruise, massaging it in very gently.

Calendula Ointment

Calendula ointment* should be applied to the skin before you put on the arnica tincture, or the comfrey tincture compresses described below.

Comfrey Root Tincture Compresses

Comfrey root tincture* compresses are another good remedy for bruises.

Apply some calendula ointment* first so that the alcohol in the tincture doesn't draw the natural oils out of your skin. Then moisten a large wad of cotton wool with the tincture, place it over the bruise and bind it gently into place with a clean linen cloth or a bandage.

Cow Parsnip Compresses

Wash some freshly-picked cow parsnip leaves and crush them to a pulp on a wooden chopping board using a rolling pin. Apply the fresh pulp to the bruise and cover it with a warm linen cloth. If you wish you can also use whole leaves in making these compresses but remember to wash them first.

St John's Wort Oil

Apply St John's wort oil* directly to the bruise several times a day, massaging it in gently.

St John's Wort Tea

Drink two cups of St John's wort tea* every day, taking care to sip it slowly.

Swedish Bitters Compresses

Apply some calendula ointment* before you put the compress on. This will prevent the alcohol in the bitters from drawing the natural oils out of your skin. Then moisten a suitably large wad of cotton wool with Swedish bitters* and place it over the bruise, covering it with a layer of dry cotton wool to keep in the warmth, plus a layer of plastic film to protect your clothes, and bind everything gently into place with a warm cloth. Leave the compress on for four hours. Alternatively, you can apply it in the evening before going to sleep and leave it on overnight.

When you remove the compress it's advisable to dust your skin with talcum powder to prevent possible itching and irritation.

BURNS

Calendula Ointment

Melt 8 oz (250g) of pure lard in a saucepan and add two generous handfuls of calendula leaves, flowers and stems. Proceed according to the standard calendula ointment* recipe. Apply the ointment directly to the burn, very gently and carefully.

St John's Wort Oil

Apply St John's wort oil* directly to the burn, very gently and carefully. Do remember that this is only a first-aid measure — you should have the burn treated by a doctor as soon as possible!

Swedish Bitters

According to Dr Samst's old manuscript, Swedish bitters* is also an excellent remedy for burns. Moisten the burn with the bitters at regular intervals; this takes the heat out of the wound, prevents the formation of blisters and helps to promote rapid healing.

Home Remedy

Moisten a clean linen cloth with the white of a fresh egg and apply it directly to the wound. Do remember once again that this is only a first-aid measure — you should still have the burn treated by a doctor as soon as possible!

CHILBLAINS

Calamus Root Wash

This wash is a good remedy for frostbite, chilblains and also for cold hands and feet. Soak 4 oz (100g) of calamus root in 4 pt (2½l) of cold water for twelve hours. Then heat up the infusion gently, strain it and bathe the affected areas in the lukewarm liquid for a good twenty minutes.

Calendula Ointment

Calendula ointment* should be applied to the chilbains several times a day.

Mistletoe Berry Ointment

Mistletoe berries should be collected between the beginning of October and the end of December. Blend the berries with a quantity of pure lard in a procelain bowl. Apply this ointment to the affected areas in the evening before you go to sleep, and leave it on overnight. Caution: Mistletoe berries are highly poisonous and should not be taken internally.

Swedish Bitters Compresses

Chilblains and frostbite on the hands and feet can also be treated with Swedish bitters* compresses. Apply some lard or calendula ointment before putting the compress on to prevent the alcohol in the bitters from drawing the natural oils out of your skin. Then moisten a wad of cotton wool with Swedish bitters and place it over the affected area, binding it into place with a bandage or a linen cloth. Change the compress several times a day. It's also helpful to apply a Swedish bitters compress in the evening before going to sleep and to leave it on overnight.

Walnut Leaf Baths

Another way of healing chilblains is to take walnut leaf baths. Use the standard recipe for walnut leaf wash* and add the liquid to your bathwater.

Walnut Leaf Wash

Pour 1 pt (½l) of hot water into a bowl containing two heaping teaspoons of finely-chopped walnut leaves and let them steep for a while before straining them off. Use the liquid to bathe the affected areas.

CIRCULATION (poor)

Comfrey Baths

Soak a bucketful of fresh comfrey or 1 lb (500g) of dried comfrey leaves in cold water for twelve hours. Then heat the infusion up gently, and strain the liquid into your bathwater. It is important that your heart should not be below the water level. Stay in the bath for twenty minutes, and don't dry yourself off when you get out; put on a robe and get straight into bed. Stay there for an hour so that you work up a good sweat.

Hawthorn Tea

Drink two cups of hawthorn tea* in the course of the day, taking care to sip it slowly.

Hawthorn Tincture

Take between four and ten drops of hawthorn tincture* a day.

Nettle Baths

It is important that your heart should be above the water level. Stay in the nettle bath* for twenty minutes, and don't dry yourself off when you get out; put on a robe and get straight into bed. Stay there for an hour so that you work up a good sweat.

Nettle Footbaths

Soak a bucketful of fresh stinging nettle stalks and leaves in cold water for twelve hours, then heat up the infusion gently and add it to your footbath water without straining off the nettles. Bathe your feet for twenty minutes.

Nettle Wash

Using the nettle footbath recipe, bathe the affected parts of your body (e.g. the area around the heart if the circulation in your coronary arteries is poor), massaging the area gently as you do so.

Swedish Bitters Compresses

Apply some lard or calendula ointment* before you put on the compress to prevent the alcohol in the Swedish bitters* from drawing the natural oils out of your skin. Then moisten a suitably large wad of cotton wool with Swedish bitters and bind it into position with a bandage or a clean linen cloth. You can leave the compress on for between two and four hours.

CIRCULATORY SYSTEM (disorders of)

Mistletoe Tea

Mistletoe is a wonderful medicinal herb for treating all kinds of heart complaints and circulatory disorders. Amazingly enough, it normalizes both high and low blood-pressure. Drink three cups of mistletoe tea* a day, taking care to sip it slowly. It's a good idea to keep your day's supply in a pre-warmed thermos.

Swedish Bitters

Swedish bitters* helps to purify the blood and improve the circulation. As a preventive measure, take a teaspoon of bitters every morning and evening in a little lukewarm water of herb tea. You can increase the dose to anything from three teaspoons to three tablespoons a day, depending on the severity of the circulatory disorder. In the case of the larger doses it's best to dissolve each spoonful in half a cup of tea and to divide this dose into two equal portions, taking one of them before eating and the other one afterwards. Drink it very slowly, one sip at a time.

Yarrow Tea

Drink up to three cups of yarrow tea* a day, taking care to sip it slowly.

Home Remedy

Soak a small towel in cold water and then wring it out so that it is quite damp, but not dripping wet. Place the towel over your heart when you go to bed, covering it with a layer of plastic film to protect your clothes from the damp and a dry towel to retain the heat, and leave it on overnight.

It's also advisable to take a cold shower after every bath, or at least to rinse off your whole body with cold water and a washcloth. This improves the circulation and tones up the entire body.

COLDS

Chamomile Inhalations

Pour 2 pt (1l) of boiling water into a bowl containing a heaped tablespoonful of chamomile, lean over the bowl, cover your head with a towel and inhale the vapours. It's absolutely essential that you keep yourself very warm after this treatment, otherwise it will be less effective.

Meadowsweet Tea

Drink two to three cups of meadowsweet tea* in the course of the day, taking care to sip it slowly.

Nettle Tea

The stinging nettle is a wonderful plant, with many different medicinal properties. For instance, it increases the body's resistance to disease, which makes it a good preventive measure to ward off colds.

You can drink up to 3½ pt (2l) of nettle tea* a day. It's a good idea to keep your day's supply in a pre-warmed thermos.

Swedish Bitters

If you have a bad cold it helps to put a few drops of Swedish bitters* on a large spoon and to inhale the vapors for a while through your mouth and nose.

In addition to the yarrow tea described below it's also advisable to take three teaspoons of Swedish bitters every day, dissolving each teaspoonful in half a cup of the tea. Divide each of these three doses into two portions, taking one of them half an hour before eating and the other half an hour afterwards.

Yarrow Tea

Take several cups of yarrow tea* a day, drinking it as hot as possible and taking care to sip it slowly.

Home Remedy

Hot footbaths are also helpful. Make the water as hot as you can bear it and add more hot water as soon as it cools. Soak your feet for ten to fifteen minutes.

COMPLEXION (poor)

Ramsons (Broad-leaved Garlic)

The blood-purifying properties of ramsons make it an excellent choice for the treatment of a chronically poor complexion. The fresh leaves can be collected in the spring, and should be eaten raw. Wash the leaves, chop them up finely, and sprinkle them on your food, as you would fresh parsley. Spinach tastes lovely if you cook it with a few ramsons leaves, and they also make an excellent addition to salads.

Ramsons (Broad-leaved Garlic) Tincture

Drying ramsons destroys its potency, so the only way of benefiting from its wonderful healing properties all the year round is to prepare a supply of ramsons tincture.* Take between ten and fifteen drops of the tincture four times a day in a little lukewarm water.

Wild Chicory Tea

Drink one cup of wild chicory tea* every morning, taking care to sip it slowly.

CONJUNCTIVITIS

Chamomile Compresses and Eyewash

Conjunctivitis can be treated with chamomile in the form of compresses and eyewash.

To make the chamomile compress, first pour a scant ½ pt (¼l) of boiling milk into a bowl containing a heaping teaspoonful of chamomile, and let it stand for thirty seconds before straining it. Then soak a clean linen cloth in the milk and lay it over your eyes, keeping your eyelids closed.

For the chamomile eyewash, use chamomile tea* to the standard recipe. When the tea has cooled, bathe your eyes with it very gently and carefully, keeping your eyes closed as you do so.

CONSTIPATION

Club Moss Tea

A good remedy for constipation is to drink a cup of hot club moss tea* in the morning before breakfast. Sip the tea slowly, and don't drink more than one cup a day!

Cow Parsnip Tea

Drink two or three cups of cow parsnip tea* in the course of the day, taking care to sip it slowly.

Figs and Prunes

Soak some figs and prunes in cold water overnight. Warm them up gently in the morning and eat them before breakfast.

Linseed (Flax Seed)

Take three tablespoons of linseed with each meal, washing it down with a little liquid until your bowel movements have returned to normal again.

Nettle Tea

Nettle tea* also helps to regulate bowel movements. Drink one cup half an hour before breakfast in the morning and two or three more cups spread over the rest of the day. You should drink the tea very warm and unsweetened, taking care to sip it slowly.

Ramsons (Broad-leaved Garlic)

Ramsons has a regulatory effect on the digestion and is an excellent remedy for constipation.

The fresh leaves should be collected in the spring and eaten raw. Wash the leaves, chop them up finely, and sprinkle them on your food as you would fresh parsley. Spinach tastes lovely if you cook it with a few ramsons leaves, and they also make an excellent addition to salads.

Ramsons (Broad-leaved Garlic) Tincture

Drying ramsons destroys its potency, so the only way of benefiting from its wonderful healing properties all the year round is to prepare a supply of ramsons tincture.* Take between ten and fifteen drops of ramsons tincture four times a day, dissolved in a little water.

Swedish Bitters

Take three teaspoonsfuls of Swedish bitters* a day in one of the herb teas described here.

Walnut Leaf Tea

Walnut leaf tea* is yet another effective remedy for constipation. Drink one cupful every morning before breakfast, taking care to sip it slowly.

Water

A very simple way of helping your bowels along is to drink a glass of fresh well water or spring water every morning before breakfast. If the constipation or other digestive disorder continues for a long time, you should also change your diet. Cut down on all refined flour products (such as white noodles, spaghetti, cakes and pastries etc.), tinned foods, meat of all kinds (especially smoked meats, pork, sausages and potted meats), all deep-fried foods and chips, cooking oils and homogenized milk products. Eat more fruit, vegetables and foods containing a high percentage of dietary fibre.

Wild Chicory Tea

Drink between half and one cup of wild chicory tea* before breakfast, taking care to sip it slowly.

Yarrow Tea

Take two or three cups of yarrow tea* a day, drinking it as hot as possible and taking care to sip it slowly.

CONTUSIONS (painful)

Arnica Tincture

Apply arnica tincture* to the contusion several times a day.

Calendula Tincture Compresses

Calendula tincture is another effective remedy for painful contusions and crush wounds.

Dilute the tincture with boiled water (let the water cool first), moisten a clean linen cloth with the diluted tincture and lay it on the affected area. It's advisable to apply some calendula ointment* before you put the compress on to prevent the alcohol in the tincture from drawing the natural oils out of your skin.

Comfrey Tincture Compresses

Apply some calendula ointment* before you put the compress on so that the tincture doesn't draw the natural oils out of your skin. Then moisten a wad of cotton wool with comfrey root tincture,* place it over the contusion and bind it gently into place with a clean linen cloth or a bandage.

Thyme Compresses

Fill a pillowcase or cushion-cover with dried thyme, sew it shut and apply it to the contusion as a compress.

CORNS

Celandine Juice

Wash some fresh celandine leaves, stems and flowers and run them through a juice extractor. Apply the undiluted juice to the corns several times a day.

Comfrey Root Ointment

Melt 8 oz (270g) of pure lard in a saucepan. Wash four to six fresh comfrey roots, chop them finely and add them to the hot fat. Proceed according to the standard recipe for ointment.* Apply this ointment to the corns every day.

Nettle Footbaths

Soak some fresh stinging nettle stems and leaves in 1 gal (5l) of cold water for twelve hours. Then heat up the infusion gently and bathe your feet in it for twenty minutes without straining off the nettles.

Nettle Root Tincture

The stinging nettle can be used to treat corns in a variety of different ways. This nettle root tincture is an excellent external remedy. Fill a glass bottle with washed, finely-chopped spring or autumn stinging nettle roots and add enough 38-40% grain alcohol to cover them completely. Leave the sealed bottle to stand in a warm place for at least two weeks. Apply the tincture to the corns several times a day.

Nettle Tea

Drink up to four cups of nettle tea* a day, taking care to sip it slowly.

Swedish Bitters

Apply Swedish bitters* to the corns several times a day, dabbing it on gently with cotton wool. When you go to bed at night, moisten a small wad of cotton wool with Swedish bitters, position it over the corn and put on a warm sock to hold it in place overnight. When you treat corns with Swedish bitters it's important to make sure that the affected area is kept damp.

COUGHS

Coltsfoot Tea
Coltsfoot is an excellent remedy for severe coughs; it soothes the inflamed tissues and also acts as an expectorant. The yellow flowerheads can be collected in the early spring, the leaves in May. Use one heaping teaspoonful of a mixture made of equal parts of flowers and leaves for each cup of tea. Pour on hot water and let the herbs steep for thirty seconds before straining them off. Drink several cups of this tea a day as hot as you can bear it, sweetening it with a little honey.

Herbal Mixture
Mix equal parts of coltsfoot flowers and leaves, smaller mullein flowers, lungwort leaves and plantain leaves. Drink three cups of tea brewed from this mixture every day, sweetening it with a little honey. Use two heaping teaspoons of the mixture for each cup of tea, pour on hot water and let the herbs steep for thirty seconds before straining them off. Drink the tea slowly, one sip at a time.

Knotgrass Tea
Drink two cups of knotgrass tea* in the course of the day, taking care to sip it slowly.

Mallow Tea
Use one heaping teaspoonful of mallow leaves, flowers and stems for each cup of tea. Steep the herbs in the cold water for twelve hours, then strain off the mallow and heat up the infusion gently before drinking it. Drink two to three cups of mallow tea in the course of the day, taking care to sip it slowly. If you have a bad cold you can apply the strained herbs to your throat and chest as a compress, heating the mallow up over a pot of boiling water first.

Plantain Tea
Take several cups of plantain tea a day, drinking it as hot as you can bear it and taking care to sip it slowly.

Home Remedy

Pour a little milk into a saucepan (just enough to cover the bottom completely) and add 4 oz (125g) of cottage cheese. Mix the milk and the cottage cheese well and then warm them up gently on a low heat, stirring constantly. When the mixture is warm (don't let it become too hot) spread it on a clean linen cloth and lay the cloth on your chest overnight, binding it into place with another cloth (and a layer of plastic film if you wish) to protect the bedclothes.

CRADLE CAP

Chamomile Tea
Give the child three to four cups of chamomile tea* in the course of the day. You can also use the tea for bathing the affected area.

Oak Bark Wash
Soak 4 oz (100g) of oak bark (available at health food stores) in 1 gal (5l) of cold water for twelve hours, then heat up the infusion gently and strain it. Bathe the affected areas with the liquid.

Walnut Leaf Wash
Bathing the affected areas with a walnut leaf wash* brings rapid relief.

CRAMPS

Chamomile Tea
The healing properties of the chamomile flower are of great help when it comes to dealing with painful cramps, especially where the patients are small children. Drink one or two cups of chamomile tea* a day, taking care to sip it slowly.

Club Moss Compresses
A good remedy for severe cramps is to bind a handful of dried club moss shoots on to the affected area with a clean linen cloth.

Meadowsweet Tincture
Take between ten and fifteen drops of meadowsweet tincture every day.

Mistletoe Tea
Mistletoe tea is a good remedy for chronic cramps.

Drink up to three cups a day (depending on the severity of the cramps) and take care to sip it slowly. It's a good idea to keep your day's supply in a pre-warmed thermos.

Sage Tea
Drink two cups of sage tea* a day, taking care to sip it slowly.

Swedish Bitters
Swedish bitters* are also useful for the treatment of severe cramps in the hands and feet, which can sometimes be crippling. Take a total of three tablespoons of the bitters every day, dissolving each tablespoonful in half a cup of lukewarm water or herb tea. Divide each of these three doses into two portions, taking one before eating and the other one afterwards.

Thyme Compresses
Thyme is a good remedy for all kinds of cramps, and especially for stomach cramps, period cramps and other abdominal cramps.

To make a thyme compress, fill a pillowcase or cushion-cover with dried thyme flowers and stems and apply it directly to the affected area. A particularly effective way of applying these compresses is to warm them up in the oven first (use the lowest setting). It's a good idea to put the compress on before you go to bed in the evening and to leave it on all night.

Thyme Tea
Drink two cups of thyme tea* in the course of the day, making sure that you sip it slowly.

CRAMPS (in the calves)

Club Moss Compresses
Fill a pillowcase or cushion cover with 3 to 9 oz (100–300g) of club moss (vary the quantity according to the size of the pillowcase) and apply it to the cramped muscle overnight.

CUTS

Lady's Mantle
Wash some fresh lady's mantle and then crush it to a pulp on a wooden chopping board using a rolling pin. Apply the fresh pulp directly to the cut.

Plantain Leaves
Wash some fresh plantain leaves and crush them to a pulp on a wooden chopping board using a rolling pin. Apply the fresh pulp directly to the cut.

Swedish Bitters
If you apply a little Swedish bitters* to a cut with a small wad of cotton wool, repeating this up to forty times at regular intervals, you will find that it will heal without leaving any scars, just as Dr. Samst claims in the old manuscript in which the recipe for the bitters was found.

CYSTITIS

Deadnettle Sitz Baths
Soak 4 oz (100g) of deadnettles in 8 pt (5l) of cold water for twelve hours, then heat the infusion up gently and strain it into your bathwater. The water should be just deep enough to cover your kidneys. Stay in the bath for twenty minutes, and don't dry yourself off when you get out; put on a robe and get straight into bed. Stay there for an hour so that you work up a good sweat.

In addition to taking the sitz baths you should also have one cup of deadnettle tea* every day. Drink it slowly, one sip at a time.

Horsetail Vapor Baths
Place a bowl containing four teaspoons of horsetail on the floor and pour on 2 pt (1l) of very hot water. Put on a robe and squat over the bowl, letting the horsetail vapors work on your bladder for ten minutes. You can also use the strained-off horsetail to make a warm poultice, wrapping it in a clean linen cloth and placing it over your bladder.

Maize Tassel Tea
Take one tablespoonful of maize tassel tea* every two to three hours. It's a good idea to keep your day's supply in a pre-warmed thermos.

DANDRUFF

Horsetail Rinse
An effective way of dealing with dandruff is to use this horsetail rinse once a day and to follow this with a scalp massage using good-quality olive oil.

Pour 2 pt (1l) of hot water into a bowl containing four heaping teaspoons of horsetail and let it steep for thirty seconds before straining it. Rinse your hair thoroughly with the liquid, rubbing it in well, and don't wash it out with water afterwards. Massage your scalp with the olive oil while your hair is still wet.

Nettle Rinse
Pour 1 pt (½l) of hot water into a bowl containing two heaping teaspoonfuls of stinging nettles and let them steep for thirty seconds before straining them off. Wash your hair with one half of the liquid, using Castile soap instead of shampoo, and rinse out the soap with the other half. Don't rinse out your hair with water afterwards. Repeat the process once a week.

DEPRESSION

Herbal Mixture
Mix equal parts of stinging nettles, yarrow and horsetail. Drink two cups of tea brewed from this mixture every day, one in the morning and one in the evening. Use one heaping teaspoonful of the mixture for each cup of tea, pour on hot water and let the herbs steep for thirty seconds before straining them off. Drink the tea slowly, one sip at a time.

Horsetail Sitz Baths
Soak 4 oz (100g) of dried horsetail (the great horsetail is best for this purpose) in cold water for twelve hours. Then heat up the infusion gently until it is almost boiling, and strain the the liquid into your bathwater. The water should be just deep enough to cover your kidneys. Stay in the bath for twenty minutes, and don't dry yourself off when you get out; put on a robe and get straight into bed. Stay there for an hour so that you work up a good sweat.

St John's Wort Tea
Drink between two and three cups of St John's wort tea* a day, taking care to sip it slowly.

St John's Wort Sitz Baths
The St John's Wort sitz bath* should be just deep enough to cover your kidneys. Stay in the bath for twenty minutes, and don't dry yourself off when you get out; put on a robe and get straight into bed. Stay there for an hour so that you work up a good sweat. It's advisable to take one of these sitz baths every week and one St John's wort footbath a day on the other six days.

Swedish Bitters
Take three tablespoons of Swedish bitters* every day, dissolving each spoonful in half a cup of herb tea. Divide each of these three doses into two portions, taking one before eating and the other one afterwards.

Thyme Baths
It is important that your heart should be above the water level. Stay in the thyme bath* for twenty minutes, and don't dry yourself off when you get out; put on a robe and get straight into bed. Stay there for an hour so that you work up a good sweat.

Wild Chicory Root Tea
Use one heaping teaspoonful of wild chicory root for each cup of tea and soak it in the cold water for twelve hours. Then heat up the infusion gently and strain it. Drink two cups of this tea in the course of the day, taking care to sip it slowly. It's a good idea to keep your day's supply in a pre-warmed thermos so that you don't need to heat it up again every time you drink it.

DIARRHOEA

Calamus Root Tea
Don't drink more than one cup of calamus root tea* a day, taking one mouthful before and after each meal. Warm the tea up gently in a water bath before drinking it.

Calendula Tea
Drink two cups of calendula tea* in the course of the day, taking care to sip it slowly.

Chamomile Tea
Drink three cups of chamomile tea* during the day, sipping it slowly.

Knotgrass Tea
Drink two cups of knotgrass tea* in the course of the day, making sure that you sip it slowly.

Ramsons (Broad-leaved Garlic)
In addition to purifying the blood, ramsons is also very useful for the treatment of all kinds of gastro-intestinal disorders.

Fresh ramsons leaves should be collected in the spring and eaten raw. Wash the leaves, chop them up finely, and sprinkle them on your food as you would fresh parsley. Spinach tastes lovely if you cook it with a few ramsons leaves, and they also make an excellent addition to salads.

Ramsons (Broad-leaved Garlic) Tincture

Drying ramsons destroys its potency, so the only way of benefiting from its wonderful healing properties all the year round is to prepare a supply of ramsons tincture.* Take between ten and fifteen drops of ramsons tincture four times a day, dissolved in a little water.

DISLOCATED JOINTS

See Sprains.

DYSMENORRHOEA (period pains)

Chamomile Tea

The unassuming and yet multi-talented chamomile is a useful remedy for period pains, and also for irregular or missed periods. Drink up to three cups of chamomile tea* a day, taking care to sip it slowly.

Deadnettle Tea

Drink two cups of deadnettle tea* a day, taking care to sip it slowly.

Herbal Mixture

Mix 1 oz (25g) of arnica blossoms, 2 oz (50g) of valerian root, 1 oz (25g) of Icelandic moss, 1 oz (25g) of lemon balm, 1 oz (25g) of sage, 1 oz (25g) of yarrow. A tea brewed from this herbal mixture is an excellent remedy for excessive menstrual bleeding.

Mix the herbs very well, and use one heaped teaspoonful of the mixture for each cup of tea. Pour on hot water and let the herbs steep for thirty seconds before straining them off. Drink one cup of the tea every morning before breakfast. It's advisable to go on drinking this tea for quite a while, even when your periods have returned to normal.

Knotgrass Tea

Drink two cups of knotgrass tea* a day, taking care to sip it slowly.

Lady's Mantle Tea

Lady's mantle is a good remedy for all sorts of menstrual disorders. Drink two to three cups of lady's mantle tea* every day, taking care to sip it slowly.

For menstrual disorders during puberty it's advisable to take a tea brewed from a mixture of equal parts of lady's mantle and yarrow. Use one heaped teaspoonful of the mixture for each cup of tea. Pour on hot water and let the herbs steep for thirty seconds before straining them off. Drink two to three cups a day, sipping it slowly.

Mistletoe Tea

Mistletoe tea* is a good treatment for all complaints that have to do with the heart and circulatory system, which makes it useful in treating menstrual disorders as well. Depending on the severity of the condition, you can drink up to three cups of this tea a day, taking care to sip it slowly. It's a good idea to keep your day's supply in a pre-warmed thermos.

Shepherd's Purse Tea

Shepherd's purse tea* is an effective treatment for excessive menstrual bleeding. You should start to take the tea eight to ten days before your period is due, drinking two cups every day until it starts. Drink it slowly, one sip at a time.

Shepherd's purse tea is also useful for normalizing irregular periods during puberty.

Swedish Bitters

Dr. Samst's old manuscript in which the recipe for Swedish bitters* was found also mentions that they can be used for treating missed periods and excessive menstrual bleeding. For three days during your period take three teaspoons of bitters a day in a little water or herb tea, and repeat this treatment every month until your periods have returned to normal.

Thyme Compresses

Thyme compresses can bring relief from period cramps. Fill a large pillowcase with dried thyme flowers and stems and apply it to your lower abdomen as a compress when you go to bed at night.

Thyme Tea

Thyme tea* helps to normalize irregular periods. Drink two cups a day, taking care to sip it slowly.

Wild Chicory Tea

Drink one cup of wild chicory tea* every morning, taking care to sip it slowly.

Yarrow Tea

Yarrow tea* is helpful in treating missed periods and irregular periods during puberty. Drink one cup of the tea every day before breakfast.

EARS (ringing in)

Cranesbill Tincture
Dab a little cranesbill tincture* into your ears with a small wad of cotton wool several times a day.

Hawthorn Tea
Drink two cups of hawthorn tea* in the course of the day, taking care to sip it slowly.

Hawthorn Tincture
Take between four and ten drops of hawthorn tincture* a day.

Mistletoe Tea
Ringing in the ears is often a symptom of high blood-pressure and concentration of the blood in the head. In these cases mistletoe's ability to regulate the action of the entire circulatory system can be of great help. Drink two to three cups of mistletoe tea* a day, taking care to sip it slowly. It's a good idea to keep your day's supply in a pre-warmed thermos. **(N.B. Do not use mistletoe berries.)**

Swedish Bitters
Another quick and effective way of dealing with ringing in the ears is to soak a little wad of cotton wool in Swedish bitters* and place it in your ear. It's a good idea to put in a few drops of warm oil or a little calendula ointment* first, as the alcohol in the bitters draws the natural oils out of the skin.

Home Remedy

Soak a small towel in cold water and then wring it out so that it is quite damp, but not dripping wet. Place the towel over your heart when you go to bed, covering it with a layer of plastic film to protect your clothes from the damp and a dry towel to keep the warmth in, and leave it on overnight.

EARACHE

Coltsfoot Juice
Wash some freshly-picked coltsfoot leaves, run them through a juice extractor, and put a few drops of the juice in your ear with a dropper.

Swedish Bitters
Moisten a small wad of cotton wool with Swedish bitters* and put it in your ear. It's advisable to apply a little warm oil or calendula ointment* to the inside of your ear beforehand so that the alcohol in the Swedish bitters doesn't draw the natural oils out of your skin and cause itching.

ECZEMA

Nettle Tea
Drink up to four cups of nettle tea* during the day, taking care to sip it slowly.

Speedwell and Nettle Tea
Mix equal quantities of speedwell and fresh stinging nettle tips. Use one heaped teaspoonful of this mixture for each cup of tea. Pour on hot water and let the herbs steep for thirty seconds before straining them off. Drink two cups of this tea every day, making sure that you sip it slowly.

EXHAUSTION

Chamomile baths
Pour some hot water into a large bowl containing four handfuls of chamomile flowers and let them steep for a while.. Then strain off the chamomile and add the liquid to your bathwater. It is important that your heart should be above the water level. Stay in the bath for twenty minutes, and don't dry yourself off when you get out; put on a robe and get straight into bed. Stay there for an hour so that you work up a good sweat.

Nettle Tea
Exhaustion, fatigue and decreased performance are often symptoms of an iron deficiency. Stinging nettles contain iron and are an effective remedy for iron deficiencies. A four-week course of treatment with nettle tea can work wonders. (The best time for this is the spring or the autumn, when you can use fresh nettles.)

Use a handful of fresh stinging nettle leaves and stalks for each cup of tea. Pour on hot water and let the nettles steep for thirty seconds before straining them off. Take care to drink the tea slowly, one sip at a time.

Drink the first cup of tea early in the morning, half an hour before eating breakfast and two more cups during the day. It's a good idea to keep your day's supply in a pre-warmed thermos.

EYEACHE

Arnica Tincture
Apply a few drops of arnica tincture* to your eyelids

and very carefully to the skin around the corners of your eyes several times a day, keeping your eyes closed as you do so. Take care not to use arnica tincture on broken skin.

Calamus Root Juice

Fresh calamus root juice can help to strengthen weak eyes. Wash the roots very carefully and run them through a juice extractor without drying them. You can apply this juice to your closed eyelids several times a day, rinsing it off with fresh water after a few minutes.

Chamomile Compresses

Pour ½ pt (¼l) of boiling milk into a bowl containing a heaped teaspoonful of chamomile and let it steep for half a minute before straining it. Let the milk cool until it is hand-hot, then soak a clean linen cloth in it and lay the cloth over your closed eyes.

Swedish Bitters

The effect of Swedish bitters* is similar to that of arnica tincture. Apply a few drops of Swedish bitters to your eyelids with your index finger twice a day (once in the early morning and once in the evening), spreading it from the bridge of your nose outwards towards the corners of your eyes. Keep your eyes closed while you are doing this.

Swedish Bitters Compresses

Swedish bitters* compresses are an excellent way of soothing overworked and strained eyes. Moisten two pads of cotton wool with Swedish bitters and then lie down and place them over your closed eyes, leaving them there for an hour. Do not apply these compresses more than once a day.

Yarrow Tea

Yarrow tea* is a good remedy for watering eyes combined with stabbing eye pains. Drink one to two cups of this tea in the course of the day, taking care to sip it slowly.

EYESIGHT (weak)

Arnica Tincture

Arnica tincture* can help to improve weak eyesight. Apply the tincture to the skin around the corners of your eyes and to your eyelids several times a day, keeping your eyes closed.

Calamus Root Juice

Scrub some fresh calamus roots thoroughly with

a brush under running water and run the wet roots through a juice extractor. Apply the fresh juice to your closed eyes several times a day, leaving it on for a few minutes before rinsing it off again with fresh, cold water. It won't be long before you start to notice that your eyesight is improving.

Calendula Tea

You can use calendula tea* as an eyewash. Pour some of the lukewarm tea into an eyeglass (you can buy one at any chemist's) and bathe your eyes with it.

Swedish Bitters

Swedish bitters* can also help to improve weak eyesight. Soak a cloth in diluted Swedish bitters and lay it over your eyes, leaving it there for an hour. Repeat this treatment every day.

In addition to this you should also apply a little Swedish bitters to your eyelids twice a day, once in the morning and once in the evening. Apply it with your fingers, stroking it outwards from the bridge of your nose towards the corners of your eyes.

FAINTING

Swedish Bitters

Swedish bitters* are a good first-aid measure for fainting. Give the patient a tablespoonful of the bitters dissolved in a little water or herb tea. Lift up their head, open their mouth and administer the liquid very slowly with a small spoon.

FATIGUE

Herbal Sitz Baths

A mixture made of equal parts of golden rod, lemon balm, field horsetail and thyme make a perfect bath tincture for treating fatigue. Steep 3 oz (85g) of the herbs in 1 gal (5l) of cold water for twelve hours, and then heat the infusion up gently, sieve off the herbs and add the liquid to your bathwater. The water should be only just deep enough to cover your lower back. Stay in the bath for twenty minutes, and don't dry yourself off when you get out; put on a robe and get straight into bed. Stay there for an hour so that you work up a good sweat.

Swedish Bitters

People whose jobs force them to travel a great deal and to take part in demanding conferences and long discussions and meetings often feel exhausted and drained. Swedish bitters* are a very good remedy for this kind of fatigue, reviving flagging spirits very rapidly. Dissolve some Swedish bitters in a little water and dab it on to your forehead, temples, closed eyelids and behind your ears. You'll be surprised how quickly this revives you, and I'm sure that you'll agree with me that it's a good idea to take a small bottle of Swedish bitters with you whenever you go on a journey.

FEET (cold)

Calamus Root Footbaths
Soak 4 oz (100g) of calamus root in cold water for twelve hours. Then heat the infusion up gently and let it steep for five minutes before straining the liquid into the water for your footbath. Bathe your feet for twenty minutes.

FEET (cramps in)

Club Moss Compresses
Cramps in the feet and calves can be treated with club moss compresses. Fill a pillowcase with 4 to 8 oz (100-200g) of dried club moss (depending on the size of the cramped muscle), apply it to the affected area and leave it on overnight.

FEET (sore and chafed)

Butterbur Leaf Dressings
Wash some fresh butterbur leaves, crush them to a pulp on a wooden chopping board using a rolling pin and apply the pulp to your feet. For speedy relief it's best to repeat this procedure several times a day.

Plantain Leaf Dressings
Wash some fresh plantain leaves, crush them to a pulp on a wooden chopping board using a rolling pin and apply the pulp to your feet. Again, it's best to repeat this procedure several times a day.

FEET (sweaty)

Horsetail Footbaths
A daily horsetail footbath can make the application of horsetail tincture (see below) unnecessary. Soak 4 oz (100g) of horsetail in cold water for twelve hours, then heat up the infusion gently and strain it into the water for your footbath. Bathe your feet for twenty minutes every day.

Horsetail Tea
Drink one cup of horsetail tea* every day before breakfast, taking care to sip it slowly.

Horsetail Tincture
This is an excellent external remedy for sweaty feet. Fill a glass bottle with fresh horsetail and add enough 38-40% grain alcohol to cover it completely. Leave the sealed bottle to stand in a warm place for at least two weeks. Wash and dry your feet thoroughly and then apply the tincture with a wad of cotton wool.

Walnut Leaf Footbaths
Pour 2 pt (1l) of hot water into a bowl containing four heaping teaspoons of finely-chopped walnut leaves and let them steep for thirty seconds before straining them off and adding the liquid to the water for your footbath. Soak your feet in this mixture for twenty minutes.

FEET (swollen)

Coltsfoot Footbaths
Pour hot water into a bowl containing two handfuls of fresh coltsfoot leaves and let them steep for two minutes before straining the liquid into the water for your footbath. Soak your feet for twenty minutes.

Mallow Footbaths
Soak two handfuls of fresh mallow leaves in 1 gal (5l) of cold water for twelve hours, then heat the infusion up gently and strain the liquid into the water for your footbath. Bathe your feet for twenty minutes.

FEVER

Chamomile tea
Drink two to three cups of chamomile tea* during the day (depending on how high your temperature is), taking care to sip it slowly.

Coltsfoot Root Tea
Use one heaping teaspoonful of coltsfoot root for each cup of tea and soak it in the cold water for twelve hours, then strain off the coltsfoot. Drink

one or two cups of this tea during the day (depending on the severity of the fever), taking care to sip it slowly.

Lady's Mantle Tea
Drink two to three cups of lady's mantle tea* a day, making sure that you sip it slowly.

Home Remedy
Before going to sleep in the evening, put on a pair of socks moistened with vinegar water and leave them on overnight. Alternatively, you can moisten two clean cloths with vinegar water and wrap them around your calves.

Swedish Bitters
In addition to the tea it's a good idea to take one to three tablespoons of Swedish bitters* a day, depending on how high the fever is. Dissolve each tablespoonful in half a cup of herb tea and divide each dose into two portions, taking one of them half an hour before eating and the other half an hour afterwards.

FLATULENCE

Calamus Root Tea
Drink one mouthful of calamus root tea* before and after each meal, i.e. a total of six mouthfuls a day. This is equivalent to one cup, and it is important not to drink more than this quantity in any one day. It's a good idea to keep your day's supply in a pre-warmed thermos. If you don't have a thermos, you can heat the tea up gently in a water bath.

Chamomile Tea
Drink a cup of chamomile tea* slowly, one sip at a time.

Sage Tea
Drink two cups of sage tea* a day, taking care to sip it slowly.

Yarrow Tea
Drink a cup of yarrow tea* slowly, one sip at a time.

FRECKLES

Bedstraw Ointment
Bedstraw ointment is very effective in treating unsightly freckles. Melt 1 lb (500g) of pure lard in

a saucepan and add four generous handfuls of bedstraw. Proceed according to the standard recipe for ointment.*

Bedstraw Wash
Bathe the affected area with a bedstraw wash* every day.

Calendula Juice
Wash the stems of some freshly-picked calendula plants and run them through a juice extractor. Apply this juice to the affected area several times a day.

Cedar Tincture
Apply cedar tincture* to the affected areas several times a day, using a wad of cotton wool.

Houseleek Sap
Take some fresh houseleek leaves, wash them, cut them into long thin strips and, using your fingers, gently apply the sap which they exude to the affected areas.

Nettle Tea
Drink up to four cups of nettle tea* a day, taking care to sip it slowly.

FUNGAL INFECTIONS (vaginal)

Calendula Sitz Baths
Vaginal fungal infections can be healed with the help of calendula sitz baths. Soak 4 oz (100g) of calendula in 1 gal (5l) of cold water for twelve hours. Then heat up the infusion gently and strain the liquid into your bathwater. The water should be just deep enough to cover your kidneys. Stay in the bath for twenty minutes, and don't dry yourself off when you get out; put on a robe and get straight into bed. Stay there for an hour so that you work up a good sweat.

GALL-BLADDER COMPLAINTS

Swedish Bitters
Gall-bladder complaints, which are often caused by rich, greasy foods, can be treated effectively with Swedish bitters.* Take one tablespoonful of

Swedish bitters twice a day (morning and evening) in a little lukewarm water or herb tea.

Swedish Bitters Compresses
In the case of stubborn gallbladder complaints it's helpful to apply a Swedish bitters* compress in the evening before going to sleep and to leave it on overnight. Apply some lard or calendula ointment* before putting on the compress to keep the alcohol in the bitters from drawing the natural oils out of your skin. Then moisten a suitably large wad of cotton wool with Swedish bitters and place it over the painful area, binding it into place with a bandage or a linen cloth.

GASTRITIS

Mallow Tea
Drink up to four cups of mallow tea in the course of the day, taking care to sip it slowly.

Swedish Bitters
Take between two and three tablespoons of Swedish bitters* a day (depending on the severity of the gastritis). Dissolve each tablespoonful in half a cup of herb tea and divide each of these doses into two portions, taking one half an hour before eating and the other half an hour afterwards.

GIDDINESS

Hawthorn Tea
Drink two cups of hawthorn tea* in the course of the day, taking care to sip it slowly.

Hawthorn Tincture
Take between four and ten drops of hawthorn tincture* every day.

Mistletoe Tea
Drink three cups of mistletoe tea* every day, taking care to sip it slowly. It's a good idea to keep your day's supply in a pre-warmed thermos.

Ramsons (Broad-leaved Garlic)
The fresh leaves should be collected in the spring and eaten raw. Wash the leaves, chop them up finely, and sprinkle them on your food as you would fresh parsley. Spinach tastes lovely if you cook it with a few ramsons leaves, and they also make an excellent addition to salads.

Ramsons (Broad-leaved Garlic) Tincture
Drying ramsons destroys its potency, so the only way of benefiting from its wonderful healing properties all the year round is to prepare a supply of ramsons tincture*. Take between ten and fifteen drops of ramsons tincture four times a day, dissolved in a little water.

Speedwell Tea
Drink one cup of speedwell tea* in the evening before going to sleep, taking care to sip it slowly.

Swedish Bitters
Swedish bitters* are also a good remedy for giddiness, both taken internally and applied externally.

Take one teaspoonful of Swedish bitters three times a day in a little lukewarm water or herb tea. In some cases inhaling the vapours from the open bottle several times a day will do the trick. You can also sniff up a couple of drops of Swedish bitters into your nostrils, very slowly and gently, from a teaspoon.

For external application, dilute some Swedish bitters with a little water, dip a clean cloth in this liquid and lay it on your forehead. It also helps to dampen the crown of your head with the cloth.

Yarrow Tea
Take between one and two cups of yarrow tea* a day, drinking it as hot as possible and taking care to sip it slowly.

Home Remedy

Soak a small towel in cold water and then wring it out so that it is quite damp but not dripping wet. Place the towel over your heart when you go to bed, covering it with a layer of plastic film to protect your clothes and a dry towel to keep the warmth in. Leave it on overnight.

GOUT

Bracken Compresses
Separate some fresh bracken fronds from their stems, apply them to the affected area and bind them into place with a clean towel. It's best to apply this compress in the evening before you go to sleep and to leave it on all night.

Butterbur Root Tea
Drink up to two cups of butterbur root tea* a day, taking care to sip it slowly.

Calamus Root Tea

Drink one mouthful of calamus root tea* before and after each meal, i.e. a total of six mouthfuls a day. This is equivalent to one cup, and it is important not to drink more than this quantity in any one day. It's a good idea to keep your day's supply in a pre-warmed thermos. If you don't have a thermos, you can heat the tea up gently in a water bath.

Club Moss Tea

Drink one cup of club moss tea in the morning before breakfast, taking care to sip it slowly.

Comfrey Baths

Soak 8 oz (200g) of comfrey root in 1 gal (5l) of cold water for twelve hours. Then heat up the infusion gently and strain it into your bathwater. It's important that your heart should be above the water level. Stay in the bath for twenty minutes and don't dry yourself off when you get out; put on a robe and get straight into bed. Stay there for an hour so that you work up a good sweat.

Cowslip Tea

Drink one or two cups of cowslip tea* a day, taking care to sip it slowly.

Dandelion Stems

The dandelion's blood-purifying properties make it an excellent remedy for gout. Eat up to ten raw, freshly-picked dandelion stems every day, washing them carefully beforehand and chewing them very thoroughly. Don't cut off the flowers until after you have washed them. This treatment is only possible in the spring, as the dandelions must be picked while they are in flower.

Horsetail Tea

Drinking a cup of horsetail tea* every day helps to prevent rheumatism, gout and neuralgia. Drink it slowly, one sip at a time.

Maize Tassel Tea

Take one tablespoonful of maize tassel tea* every two to three hours.

Meadowsweet Tea

Drink up to three cups of meadowsweet tea* in the course of the day, taking care to sip it slowly.

Nettle Baths

Pour about 8 pt (5l) of hot water into a large bowl containing 8 oz (200g) of stinging nettles and let them steep for thirty seconds before straining the liquid into your bathwater. It's important that your heart should be above the water level. Stay in the bath for twenty minutes and don't dry yourself off when you get out; put on a robe and get straight into bed. Stay there for an hour so that you work up a good sweat.

Speedwell Tincture

Chop up two generous handfuls of flowering speedwell finely and put it in a glass bottle. Add 2 pt (1l) of 38-40% grain alcohol, seal the bottle and leave it to stand in a warm place for at least two weeks. Massage the affected areas regularly with this tincture.

It's advisable to take some speedwell tincture internally as well. Take fifteen drops three times a day in a little lukewarm water or herb tea.

Swedish Bitters

Take one teaspoonful of Swedish bitters* three times a day, dissolved in a little of one of the herb teas described above.

GUMBOILS

Bedstraw tea

Gargle with bedstraw tea* several times a day. You should also rinse the affected area with bedstraw tea every now and then.

Sage Tea

Gargle with sage tea* several times a day. As an additional measure you can soak a small wad of cotton wool in sage tea and place it against the gumboils for a while.

GUMS (bleeding)

Sage Tea

Gargle thoroughly with sage tea* several times a day. You can also soak a small wad of cotton wool in the tea and place it against the bleeding gums for a while.

Home Remedy

Dip a wet toothbrush in fresh lemon juice and massage the bleeding gums with it gently.

GUMS (inflammation of — gingivitis)

Horsetail and St John's Wort Tea

Gargle several times a day with a tea made from

equal parts of horsetail and St John's wort. Use one heaping teaspoonful of the mixture for each cup of tea. Pour on hot water and let the herbs steep for thirty seconds before straining them off. Let the tea cool before you use it.

Walnut Leaf Tea
Gargle with walnut leaf tea* several times a day.

GYNECOLOGICAL DISORDERS

Deadnettle Tea
Drink two cups of deadnettle tea* in the course of the day, taking care to sip it slowly.

Lady's Mantle Tea
Lady's mantle is a real panacea for all types of women's complaints. It's a good idea to drink lady's mantle tea* regularly as a preventive measure. Drink two to four cups of this tea a day, taking care to sip it slowly.

HEMORRHOIDS

Celandine Juice
Wash some fresh celandine leaves, stems and flowers and run them through a juice extractor. Drink the juice diluted with an equal measure of lukewarm water.

Chamomile Ointment
This is a very effective hemorrhoid ointment. Be sure to massage it in very gently.

Melt 8 oz (250g) of pure lard in a saucepan and add two generous handfuls of fresh chamomile flowers. Proceed according to the standard recipe for ointment*.

Chamomile Tea
Taken internally, chamomile is an indirect remedy for hemorrhoids, as it helps to stimulate your bowel movements without actually acting as a laxative. Drink one cup of chamomile tea* every day before breakfast, taking care to sip it slowly.

Horsetail Tea
Horsetail has the ability to staunch bleeding, which makes it a good treatment for bleeding hemorrhoids. Depending on the intensity of the bleeding use one or two heaping teaspoonfuls of

horsetail for each cup of tea. Pour on hot water and let the herbs steep for thirty seconds before straining them off. Drink two to three cups of this tea a day, taking care to sip it slowly.

Shepherd's Purse Sitz Baths
Pour hot water into a bowl containing about 4 oz (100g) of dried shepherd's purse and let the herbs steep for five minutes before straining the liquid into your bathwater. The water should be just deep enough to cover your kidneys. Stay in the bath for twenty minutes, and don't dry yourself off when you get out; put on a robe and get straight into bed. Stay there for an hour so that you work up a good sweat.

Shepherd's Purse Tea
Use lukewarm shepherd's purse tea* as a wash or as an enema.

Swedish Bitters
Moisten a wad of cotton wool with Swedish bitters* and place it against your anus, leaving it on overnight.

Take a teaspoonful of Swedish bitters before going to sleep at night, dissolving it in a little lukewarm water or herb tea.

Yarrow and Raspberry Leaf Ointment
Melt 6 oz (180g) of pure lard in a saucepan and add 1 oz (30g) of fresh, finely-chopped yarrow flowers and 1 oz (30g) of finely-chopped raspberry leaves. Proceed according to the standard recipe for ointment*. Massage the ointment into your hemorrhoids very gently.

Yarrow Tea
Yarrow tea* provides rapid relief from bleeding hemorrhoids. Drink two cups a day, one in the morning and one in the evening, taking care to sip it slowly.

HAIR (loss of)

Walnut Leaf Lotion
Pour hot water into a cup containing two heaping teaspoonfuls of finely-chopped walnut leaves and let them steep for thirty seconds before putting them through a sieve. Massage the lotion into your scalp.

Wild Chicory Juice
Fresh wild chicory juice is a good remedy for loss of eyebrow hair and eyelashes. Chew a wild chicory

stalk and apply the juice it exudes to your eyebrows and lashes with your fingers.

HAIR (unwanted)

Calendula Ointment
Calendula ointment is extremely easy to make at home. Melt 8 oz (250g) of pure lard in a saucepan and add two generous handfuls of calendula leaves, blossoms and stalks. Proceed according to the standard recipe for calendula ointment.

Chamomile Oil
Apply chamomile oil* to your entire body, massaging it in well.

Cowslip Juice
In the case of women, excess hair on fair arms and legs is usually caused by kidney dysfunctions.

This cowslip juice should always be made fresh, just before you use it. Run the stalks, flowers and leaves of freshly-picked cowslips through a juice extractor, then apply the juice, leaving it for several hours before washing it off with water and mild soap. After drying your skin it's a good idea to apply some calendula ointment, St John's wort oil or chamomile oil.

Horsetail Sitz Baths
It's helpful to take one horsetail sitz bath* a week as a supplement to a course of treatment with cowslip juice and nettle tea, as it stimulates the blood circulation in the kidneys. The horsetail sitz bath should be just deep enough to cover your kidneys. Stay in the bath for twenty minutes, and don't dry yourself off when you get out; put on a robe and get straight into bed. Stay there for an hour so that you work up a good sweat.

Nettle Tea
It's advisable to supplement the cowslip juice with at least four cups of nettle tea* a day. Drink it slowly, one sip at a time.

St John's Wort Oil
Apply St John's wort oil* all over your body, massaging it in well.

HAIR CARE

Chamomile rinse
A regular chamomile rinse will keep your hair light, fragrant and shiny. Rinse your hair with chamomile wash*, and then simply towel it dry, without washing the rinse out with water.

HAIR GROWTH (stimulation of)

Burdock Root Rinse
Soak 4 oz (100g) of burdock root in cold water for twelve hours, then heat the infusion up gently and strain it. Wash your hair with half of the liquid, using Castile soap instead of shampoo, and rinse the soap out with the other half. Don't wash the rinse out of your hair afterwards.

Hair Treatment
Put a celandine stem and equal measures (one handful each) of fresh stinging nettles, birch leaves, elderberry leaves and walnut leaves in a pot containing 8 pt (5l) of water and heat it up gently until it is almost boiling. Turn off the heat and let the herbs steep for a few minutes before straining them off. Wash your hair thoroughly with half of this liquid, using Castile soap instead of shampoo, and then rinse the soap out with fresh water. Then rinse your hair out again with the other half of the liquid, massaging it into your scalp and letting it work in for a while before towelling your hair dry. Don't wash the rinse out of your hair.

Nettle Rinse
The stinging nettle is a very underestimated plant. In addition to its many other properties, it also promotes hair growth. Put ten handfuls of fresh stinging nettles in a saucepan with 1 gal (5l) of cold water and then heat the water up gently (don't let it boil). Remove the pot from the heat and let the nettles steep for five minutes before straining them off and using the liquid for washing your hair.

An infusion made from stinging nettle roots will make your hair stronger and thicker. Soak two generous handfuls of nettle roots in cold water for twelve hours, and then heat the water up gently, remove the pot from the heat and let the roots steep for ten minutes before straining them off and washing your hair with the liquid.

Nettle Root Tincture
In addition to treating your hair with the herbal rinses described above, it's also a good idea to massage your scalp with nettle root tincture* every day. You'll find that this leaves your hair beautiful and shiny.

HALITOSIS (bad breath)

Bad breath can have many causes, and it's best that your doctor finds out exactly what the reason is in your case before you start trying to treat the symptoms. It can be caused by excretions of the mucous membranes in the nasal passages, infected tonsils, indigestion, insufficient acid in the stomach or by mouth ulcers.

Gargle with sage tea* if you have a tonsil infection, with warm bedstraw tea* or with 30-40 drops of myrrh tincture dissolved in some lukewarm water if you have mouth ulcers. You can treat nasal secretions effectively by gently sniffing a little lukewarm sage tea into the nostrils.

Bad breath can often be neutralized by taking a few drops of elderberry oil dissolved in lukewarm water: drink it slowly, one little sip at a time. Another good home remedy is to chew dill seeds. If the bad breath is caused by a furred tongue you can deal with it by taking half teaspoon of wormwood tincture dissolved in a cup of water.

HANDS (swollen)

Mallow Wash
Soak your hands in a mallow wash* for a good twenty minutes.

HAY FEVER

Nettle Tea
Drink up to four cups of nettle tea* a day, taking care to sip it slowly.

Swedish Bitters
Take three teaspoons of Swedish bitters* a day, dissolving each teaspoonful in half a cup of nettle tea. Divide each of these three doses into two portions, taking one of them before eating and the other one afterwards.

HEADACHES

Cowslip Tea
Drink up to three cups of cowslip tea* during the day, taking care to sip it slowly.

Hawthorn Tea
Drink two cups of hawthorn tea* during the day.

Hawthorn Tincture
Take between four and ten drops of hawthorn tincture* every day.

Nettle Tea
You can drink up to 3½ pt (2l) of nettle tea* a day (a cup is equivalent to about a third of a pint). It's a good idea to keep your day's supply in a pre-warmed thermos.

Swedish Bitters
If the headache is severe you can also take between two and three tablespoonfuls of Swedish bitters* a day, dissolving each spoonful in half a cup of one of the herb teas described here. Divide each of these two or three doses into two portions and take one of them before eating and the other one afterwards.

Swedish Bitters Compresses
Apply some lard or calendula ointment* to your temples and forehead before you put the compress on to prevent the alcohol in the Swedish bitters* from drawing the natural oils out of your skin. Then moisten a large wad of cotton wool with Swedish bitters and place it over your forehead, binding it into place with a bandage or a clean linen cloth. You can leave the compress on for two to four hours.

Yarrow Tea
Drink two cups of yarrow tea* a day, taking care to sip it slowly.

Home Remedy

Soak a small towel in cold water and then wring it out so that it is quite damp but not dripping wet. Place the towel over your heart when you go to bed, covering it with a layer of plastic film to protect your clothes from the damp and a dry towel to keep the warmth in, and leave it on overnight.

HEAD LICE

Walnut Leaf Wash
Not so long ago it was thought that head lice had been exterminated completely, but they now seem

to be enjoying something of a renaissance. A walnut leaf wash* is a sure way of getting rid of lice quickly. Rinse your hair with the liquid, massaging it into your scalp. Repeat this treatment every day.

HEARING (impaired)

Cranesbill Tincture
Gently apply a little cranesbill tincture* to the inside of your ears several times a day with a little wad of cotton wool.

Swedish Bitters
Before applying the Swedish bitters* it's advisable to dab a little chamomile oil* or calendula ointment* into your ears to prevent the itching that can be caused by the alcohol in the bitters. Then moisten two little wads of cotton wool with the bitters and place them in your ears. It also helps to dab a little Swedish bitters behind your ears at regular intervals.

HEARING DISORDERS

Cranesbill Tincture
Apply a little cranesbill tincture* to the inside of your ears with your finger.

Herbal Mixture
If the hearing disorder has been caused by exposure to the cold, it's advisable to rinse your ears out with a decoction made from a mixture of equal quantities of ground ivy, sage and yarrow. Place the herbs in a bowl (one heaping teaspoonful for each cup of water), pour on hot water and let the mixture steep for thirty seconds before straining it off. Let the decoction cool before you use it!

Swedish Bitters
In the old manuscript in which the recipe for Swedish bitters* was found, Dr. Samst writes that they are also a good remedy for impaired hearing. Apply a little Swedish bitters to the inside of your ear with your finger. An alternative method is to moisten a little wad of cotton wool with Swedish bitters and to place it in your ear for a while. It's advisable to put a couple of drops of warm thyme oil in your ear before applying the Swedish bitters. The easiest way to heat the oil is to put it in a teaspoon that has just been dipped in hot water.

HEARTBURN

Calendula Tea
Drink two to three cups of calendula tea* in the course of the day, taking care to sip it slowly.

Sorrel Tea
Pour 1 pt (½l) of hot water into a pot containing a tablespoonful of fresh common sorrel leaves and let them steep for thirty seconds before straining them off. Let the tea cool before you drink it. Drink two cups a day, sipping it slowly.

Yarrow Tea
Drink two or three cups of yarrow tea* a day, taking care to sip it slowly.

HICCUPS

Dill Seed Tea
This tea brings rapid relief from hiccups. Use one heaping teaspoonful of dill seeds for each cup of tea. Pour on hot water and let the herbs steep for thirty seconds before straining them off. Don't sweeten this tea and take care to drink it slowly in little sips.

HOARSENESS

Bedstraw Tea
Gargle with bedstraw tea* several times a day.

Coltsfoot Tea
Take several cups of coltsfoot tea* a day with a little honey, drinking it as hot as you can bear it and taking care to sip it slowly.

Mallow Tea
You can drink up to three cups of mallow tea* a day, depending on how hoarse you are. It's a good idea to keep your day's supply in a pre-warmed thermos.

Plantain Tea
Drink two to four cups of plantain tea* a day, taking care to sip it slowly.

IMPOTENCE

The first and most important step in the treatment of impotence is to give up cigarettes and alcohol.

Cow Parsnip Tincture
Fill a glass bottle with finely-chopped cow parsnip leaves and sprouts and add enough 38-40% grain alcohol to cover them completely. Leave the sealed bottle to stand in a warm place for at least two weeks. Take thirty drops of this tincture every day, dissolved in a little of the lady's mantle tea described below.

Lady's Mantle Tea
Drink four cups of lady's mantle tea* a day, taking care to sip it slowly.

Shepherd's Purse Tincture
Massage your lower abdomen regularly with Shepherd's purse tincture*

INDIGESTION

Agrimony Tea
Drink up to two cups of agrimony tea* a day, taking care to sip it slowly.

Comfrey Root Tea
Two to four cups of comfrey root tea* a day are an effective remedy for indigestion. It should be taken without any sugar or other sweetener. Drink the tea slowly, one sip at a time.

Cow Parsnip Tea
Drink two to three cups of cow parsnip tea* a day, taking care to sip it slowly.

Deadnettle Tea
Drink one cup of deadnettle tea* in the morning, sipping it slowly

Sorrel Tea
Drink two cups of sorrel tea* in the course of the day, taking care to sip it slowly.

Walnut Leaf Tea
Drink one to two cups of walnut leaf tea* during the day, taking care to sip it slowly.

Wild Chicory Tea
Drink one cup of wild chicory tea* in the morning, sipping it slowly.

INFECTED CUTS, etc.

Lady's Mantle Compresses
In the case of very stubborn infected cuts and grazes that heal slowly, it's helpful to supplement the effects of the tea with lady's mantle compresses. Wash four handfuls of fresh lady's mantle and crush them to a pulp on a wooden chopping board using a rolling pin. Apply the pulp directly to the wound and bind it gently into place with a clean linen cloth. Leave the compress on for a few hours, and then rinse the wound out with fresh water and repeat the whole process once.

Lady's Mantle Tea
Drink two to three cups of lady's mantle tea* a day, taking care to sip it slowly.

Sage Tea
Drink two cups of sage tea* a day, taking care to sip it slowly.

Swedish Bitters
Take between three teaspoonfuls and three tablespoonfuls of Swedish bitters* a day, depending on the severity of the diarrhea, dissolving each spoonful of bitters in half a cup of lukewarm water or herb tea. Divide each of these three doses into two portions, taking one of them half an hour before eating and the other half an hour afterwards.

INFECTIONS

Chamomile tea
Drink a cup of chamomile tea* slowly, one sip at a time.

Sage Compresses
Warm sage tea compresses are an effective treatment for infected teeth and all infections in the mouth and throat, including tonsillitis. Soak a clean cloth in warm sage tea*, wrap it around your throat and bind it into place with a clean bandage or cloth. It's also advisable to supplement this

treatment by gargling with sage tea several times a day.

Sage Tea
Drink two cups of sage tea* during the course of the day, taking care to sip it slowly.

Swedish Bitters
If the infection is severe it's a good idea to take two to three tablespoonfuls of Swedish bitters* a day, dissolving each tablespoonful in half a cup of sage tea. Divide each of these doses into two portions, taking one of them half an hour before eating and the other one half an hour afterwards.

Swedish Bitters Compresses
Apply some lard or calendula ointment* before you put on the compress to prevent the alcohol in the Swedish bitters* from drawing the natural oils out of your skin. Then moisten a wad of cotton wool with Swedish bitters and place it over the affected area, binding it into place with a bandage or a linen cloth. You can leave the compress on for between two and four hours.

INFLUENZA

Meadowsweet Tea
Drink two to three cups of meadowsweet tea* in the course of the day, taking care to sip it slowly.

Home Remedy

Take regular hot footbaths, keeping your feet in the water for ten to fifteen minutes. Make the water as hot as you can bear it, and add more hot water from time to time to keep the temperature up.

Preventive measures for influenza are listed in Chapter 2.

INJURIES IN GENERAL

Arnica Compresses
Compresses containing the arnica petals used to make arnica tincture are a very good treatment for all kind of injuries. Wrap the alcohol-soaked petals in a clean cloth and apply them directly to the injury. It's advisable to apply some calendula ointment* before you put the compress on so that

the alcohol in the tincture doesn't draw the natural oils out of your skin.

St John's Wort Oil
Injuries can also be treated with oil made from St John's wort flowers and buds. Apply the St John's wort oil* very gently to the injury and the area around it.

INSECT BITES

You can protect yourself against annoying insect bites by rubbing your skin with fresh walnut leaves.

Plantain
Wash some freshly-picked plantain leaves, crush them to a pulp on a wooden chopping board using a rolling pin and apply the pulp directly to the sting.

Sage
Take some fresh sage leaves, wash them, crush them to a pulp on a wooden chopping board using a rolling pin and apply the pulp to the sting.

Swedish Bitters
Swedish bitters* are a good first-aid remedy for stings. Moisten a small wad of cotton wool with the bitters and press it firmly on to the sting.

INSOMNIA

Chamomile Tea
Drink one cup of chamomile tea* before going to bed, taking care to sip it slowly.

Deadnettle Tea
When the insomnia is of nervous origin, relief can be obtained by drinking two cups of deadnettle tea* a day.

Hawthorn Tea
Drink two cups of hawthorn tea* in the course of the day, taking care to sip it slowly.

Hawthorn Tincture
Take between four and ten drops of hawthorn tincture* every day.

Herbal Mixture

Mix ¼ oz (5g) of valerian root, ¾ oz (15g) of hop flowers, ½ oz (10g) of St John's wort, 1¼ oz (25g) of lavender flowers and 2½ oz (50g) of cowslips. Drink a cup of tea brewed from this mixture before going to bed at night. Use one heaping teaspoonful of the mixture for each cup of tea. Pour on hot water and let the herbs steep for thirty seconds before straining them off. Drink the tea as hot as possible, taking care to sip it slowly. If you find it too bitter, you can sweeten it with a little honey.

Lady's Mantle Tea

At higher altitudes — up to 4000 ft (1300m) — one can find a variety of lady's mantle known as alpine lady's mantle. The undersides of the leaves are silvery. Tea made from these leaves brings rapid relief from insomnia. Use one heaping teaspoonful of the leaves for each cup of tea. Pour on hot water and let the herbs steep for thirty seconds before straining them off. Drink two to three cups of this tea a day, taking care to sip it slowly.

Lime Blossom Baths

When children have trouble sleeping, a lime blossom bath can work wonders.

Half fill a bucket with freshly-picked lime blossoms and soak them in cold water for twelve hours, then heat up the infusion gently and strain it into the bathwater. It's important that the child's heart should be above the water level. Let him or her stay in the bath for twenty minutes, and don't dry him or her off afterward. Instead, wrap the child up in a warm dressing gown and let him or her work up a good sweat in bed for an hour.

Meadowsweet Tea

Drink two or three cups of this tea a day, taking care to sip it slowly.

Ramsons (Broad-leaved Garlic)

Ramsons has a beneficial effect on the stomach and the rest of the digestive system and can be of help in treating insomnia caused by upset stomachs.

The fresh leaves should be collected in the spring and eaten raw. (Drying them destroys their potency.) Wash the leaves, cut them up and eat them raw. You can also chop them up finely and sprinkle them on your food, as you would fresh parsley, or you can add a few leaves to salads.

Ramsons (Broad-leaved Garlic) Tincture

Drying ramsons destroys its potency, so the only way of benefiting from its wonderful healing properties all the year round is to prepare a supply of ramsons tincture* Take between ten and fifteen drops of ramsons tincture four times a day, dissolved in a little lukewarm water.

St John's Wort Tea

Drink two to three cups of St John's wort tea* a day, taking care to sip it slowly.

St John's Wort Sitz Baths

The water in a St John's wort sitz bath* should only be just deep enough to cover your kidneys. Stay in the bath for twenty minutes and don't dry yourself off when you get out; put on a robe and get straight into bed. Stay there for an hour so that you work up a good sweat.

If you frequently suffer from insomnia, it's a good idea to take one St John's wort sitz bath and six St John's wort footbaths every week.

Home Remedy

Soak a small towel in cold water and then wring it out so that it is quite damp, but not dripping wet. Place the towel over your heart when you go to bed, covering it with a layer of plastic film to protect your clothes from the damp and a dry towel to keep the warmth in, and leave it on overnight.

Dip your arms in ice-cold water all the way up to your shoulders and count from one to twenty slowly before taking them out again. Don't dry your arms off afterwards — get straight into your pyjamas or nightgown and go to bed.

St John's Wort Tincture

Take between ten and fifteen drops of St John's wort tincture* a day, dissolving it in a tablespoonful of warm water.

Swedish Bitters

Before going to bed, take a teaspoonful of Swedish bitters* dissolved in a little of one of the herb teas described above. If the insomnia is of nervous origin, you can also moisten a clean cloth with diluted Swedish bitters and lay it over your heart as a compress before going to sleep. It's best to apply calendula ointment* to your chest beforehand to prevent the alcohol in the bitters from drawing the natural oils out of your skin.

INTESTINAL DISORDERS

Calamus Root Tea
Drink one mouthful of calamus root tea* before and after each meal, i.e., a total of six mouthfuls a day. This is equivalent to one cup, and it is important not to drink more than this quantity in any one day. Warm the tea up gently in a water bath before drinking it.

Calendula Tea
Drink three to four cups of calendula tea* in the course of a day, taking care to sip it slowly.

Mallow Tea
Drink up to three cups of mallow tea* a day, taking care to sip it slowly. It's a good idea to keep your day's supply in a pre-warmed thermos, but if you don't have a thermos, you can heat the tea up gently in a water bath before you drink it.

Sage Tea
Drink two cups of sage tea* a day, taking care to sip it slowly.

Speedwell Tea
Drink at least one cup of speedwell tea a day, taking care to sip it slowly.

Swedish Bitters
Take three teaspoons of Swedish bitters* a day, dissolving each spoonful in half a cup of one of the herb teas described above. Divide each of these doses into two portions, taking one of them before eating and the other one afterwards.

IRON DEFICIENCIES

Nettle Tea
Tea made from fresh stinging nettles helps to provide your body with the iron it needs.

Use a *handful* of fresh stinging nettles for each cup of tea. Pour on hot water and let the herbs steep for thirty seconds before straining them off. Drink two or three cups of this tea in the course of the day, taking care to sip it slowly.

IRRITABILITY AND ANGER

Chamomile Baths
A good soak in the bathtub with an infusion of chamomile in the water has a wonderfully relaxing effect on the entire nervous system. Pour hot water into a bowl containing four handfuls of chamomile flowers and let them steep for a few minutes before straining the infusion into your bathwater. It's important that your heart should be above the water level. Stay in the bath for twenty minutes, and don't dry yourself off when you get out; put on a robe and get straight into bed. Stay there for an hour so that you work up a good sweat.

Chamomile Tea
Whenever you feel yourself beginning to get annoyed or angry, make yourself a cup of chamomile tea* immediately, so that you can avoid putting a strain on your heart and circulatory system. Drink the tea slowly, one sip at a time.

Mistletoe Tea
Drink up to three cups of mistletoe tea* in the course of the day, taking care to sip it slowly.

ITCHING

Calendula ointment
Calendula ointment* is a good remedy for intense itching. Apply it to the affected area several times a day.

Dandelion
A course of treatment with fresh dandelion stems can help to alleviate irritating itching. Eat ten raw, freshly-picked dandelion stems every day, washing them carefully beforehand and chewing them very thoroughly. Don't cut off the flowers until after you have washed the plants. The dandelions must be picked while they are in flower.

Nettle Tea
Problem skin, severe bruises, allergies and rashes are all often accompanied by uncomfortable itching. The temptation to scratch is very great, but if you give in to it, it can retard the healing process. Nettle tea* can alleviate the itching. Drink up to four cups a day, taking care to sip it slowly.

Speedwell Tea

Speedwell tea* is a particularly good remedy for *pruritus senilis*, the uncomfortable itching that the elderly often suffer from. Drink up to two cups a day, taking care to sip it slowly.

Yarrow Sitz Baths

Yarrow sitz baths* and douches are a good treatment for vaginal itching. The bath water should be just deep enough to cover your kidneys. Stay in the bath for twenty minutes and don't dry yourself off when you get out; put on a robe and get straight into bed. Stay there for an hour so that you work up a good sweat. You can also use the warm infusion for vaginal douches.

JOINTS (inflammation of)

Cabbage and Club Moss Poultices

Iron some cabbage leaves (either white cabbage or savoy cabbage) until they are piping hot and apply them directly to the affected joints, binding them into place with a warm cloth.

Club moss poultices are even more effective. Take some freshly-picked club moss leaves, crush them to a pulp on a wooden chopping board using a rolling pin and apply the pulp directly to the affected joints, binding it in place with a warm cloth. It's best to apply the poultices in the evening and to leave them on overnight.

Comfrey Root Tincture

A regular gentle massage with comfrey root tincture* can help to reduce the joint pain. Massage the affected joints with this tincture every day.

Horsetail Compresses

If you suffer from inflammation of the joints, it's also advisable to apply regular hot horsetail compresses in addition to any other treatment.

Put two heaping handfuls of horsetail in a sieve and heat it up over boiling water. When the horsetail is really hot wrap it up in a clean linen cloth and apply it to the affected joint, securing it with another cloth to prevent the healing vapors from escaping and being wasted. Leave the compress on for several hours. You can use the same horsetail for making up to three compresses, heating it up again each time you use it.

Horsetail Sitz Baths

For a horsetail sitz bath* the water should be just deep enough to cover your kidneys. Stay in the bath for twenty minutes and don't dry yourself off when you get out; put on a robe and get straight into bed. Stay there for an hour so that you work up a good sweat. Take one horsetail sitz bath every month.

Horsetail Tea

Drink two cups of horsetail tea* every day, one half an hour before breakfast in the morning and the other half an hour before supper in the evening.

Nettle Tea

In addition to horsetail tea it's also a good idea to take four cups of nettle tea* a day. Drink it one sip at a time during the daytime between the two cups of horsetail tea.

Swedish Bitters

Take three tablespoons of Swedish bitters* a day, dissolving each tablespoonful in half a cup of the nettle tea*. Divide each of these three doses into two portions, taking one before eating and one afterwards.

Swedish Bitters Compresses

Apply some calendula ointment* before you put the compress on so that the alcohol in the bitters doesn't draw the natural oils out of your skin. Then moisten a large wad of cotton wool with Swedish bitters and wrap it around the joint, covering it with a layer of dry cotton wool to keep the warmth in and a layer of plastic film to protect your clothes. Bind everything into place with a clean cloth. Apply one Swedish bitters compress every day, leaving it on for four hours.

JOINTS (swollen)

Comfrey Root Tincture

The swelling can be relieved by massaging the affected joint regularly with comfrey root tincture*.

LARYNGITIS

Mallow Tea

Drink two or three cups of mallow tea* every day. It's a good idea to keep your day's supply in a pre-warmed thermos. It's also advisable to gargle with this tea several times a day, so make plenty of it in advance!

The strained-off mallow can be used in warm poultices so don't throw it away. To make a mallow poultice, heat up the herbs again and mix them with barley flour to make a paste, adding a little warm water if necessary. Apply the warm paste to a clean linen cloth and wrap it around your throat, binding it into place with another cloth. This poultice should be applied in the evening and left on all night.

LARYNGITIS (catarrhal)

Coltsfoot Tea
Drink two to three cups of coltsfoot tea* in the course of the day, taking care to sip it slowly. If you have a sweet tooth you can add a little honey.

Walnut Leaf Tea
Rinse out your mouth and throat with walnut leaf tea* several times a day.

LESIONS

Coltsfoot Dressings
Wash some freshly-picked coltsfoot leaves and crush them to a pulp on a wooden chopping board using a rolling pin. Apply this pulp directly to the lesion.

LEUCORRHEA

Horsetail Sitz Baths
A good way of treating vaginal discharge is to take one or two horsetail sitz baths* a week. The water should be just deep enough to cover your kidneys. Stay in the bath for twenty minutes and don't dry yourself off when you get out; put on a robe and get straight into bed. Stay there for an hour so that you work up a good sweat.

Knotgrass Tea
Drink two cups of knotgrass tea* during the day, making sure that you sip it slowly.

Lady's Mantle Tea
Drink up to three cups of lady's mantle tea* in the course of the day, taking small sips.

Swedish Bitters
Take three teaspoons of Swedish bitters* a day, dissolving each teaspoonful in half a cup of one of the herb teas described here. Divide each of these three doses into two portions, taking one before eating and the other one afterward.

Walnut Leaf Douche
Soak two heaping teaspoons of walnut leaves in 1 pt (½l) of cold water for twelve hours. Then heat up the infusion gently, strain off the walnut leaves and use the liquid as a vaginal douche (let it cool first).

Yarrow Sitz Baths
It's a good idea to take alternate horsetail and yarrow sitz baths*. The yarrow sitz bath should be just deep enough to cover your kidneys. Stay in the bath for twenty minutes and don't dry yourself off when you get out; put on a robe and get straight into bed. Stay there for an hour so that you work up a good sweat.

Yarrow Tea
In addition to the yarrow sitz baths it's also advisable to drink two cups of yarrow tea* every day. Drink it slowly, one sip at a time.

LUMBAGO

Agrimony Tea
Drink one or two cups of agrimony tea* a day, taking care to sip it slowly.

Meadowsweet Tea
Drink two to three cups of meadowsweet tea* a day, sipping it slowly.

St John's Wort Oil
St John's wort oil is an effective remedy for lumbago, sciatica and rheumatism: no household medicine cabinet should be without it. Massage it gently into the affected areas.

Stinging Nettles
Stroke the affected areas very gently with a freshly-picked stinging nettle. Start at the bottom and stroke upward (never downward), doing this four times in all. Then dust the reddened skin with a little talcum powder. The condition will improve after a few days of this treatment.

MELANCHOLIA

Speedwell and Celery Root Tea
This tea helps to relieve depressive moods and melancholia.

Mix equal quantities of speedwell and celery root. Use one heaping teaspoonful of the mixture for each cup of tea. Pour on hot water and let the herbs steep for thirty seconds before straining them off. Drink one cup of this tea in the evening before going to bed, taking care to sip it slowly.

MEMORY (lapses of)

Hawthorn Tea
Use one heaping teaspoonful of hawthorn leaves, flowers and berries for each cup of tea and soak them in the cold water for twelve hours. Then heat up the infusion gently and strain off the hawthorn. Drink two cups of this tea every day, taking care to sip it slowly.

Hawthorn Tincture
Take between four and ten drops of hawthorn tincture* a day.

Speedwell and Horsetail Tea
Mix equal quantities of speedwell and horsetail. Use one heaping teaspoonful of this mixture for each cup of tea. Pour on hot water and let the herbs steep for thirty seconds before straining them off. Drink two cups of this tea a day, taking care to sip it slowly.

MEMORY (poor)

Ramsons (Broad-leaved Garlic) Tincture
Ramsons tincture* can help to improve poor memory. Take between ten and twelve drops of the tincture a day, dissolved in a little water.

Speedwell Tea
Drink one cup of speedwell tea* in the evening before going to sleep, taking care to sip it slowly.

Swedish Bitters
Apply a little Swedish bitters* to the crown of your head regularly (just enough to moisten the skin).

MENOPAUSE

The menopause can be a traumatic time, with all sorts of irritating complaints suddenly appearing. The medicinal herbs from God's garden will help to make this period of your life easier to deal with and more pleasant.

Herbal Mixture
Drink one cup of tea brewed from this mixture every day before breakfast, taking care to sip it slowly.

Mix 1 oz (25g) of arnica flowers, 2 oz (50g) of valerian root, 1 oz (25g) of icelandic moss, 1 oz (25g) of lemon balm, 1 oz (25g) of yarrow and 1 oz (25g) of sage.

Use one heaping teaspoonful of the mixture for each cup of tea. Pour on hot water and let the herbs steep for thirty seconds before straining the infusion.

Lady's Mantle Tea
Drink up to three cups of lady's mantle tea* a day, sipping it slowly.

Mistletoe Tea
Drink up to three cups of mistletoe tea* in the course of the day, being careful to sip it slowly. It's a good idea to keep your day's supply in a pre-warmed thermos.

Shepherd's Purse Tea
During menopause it's a good idea to give yourself a treatment with shepherd's purse tea* at regular intervals. Drink two cups of the tea a day for four weeks. Make the two cups last the whole day, taking little sips every now and then. At the end of four weeks, leave a three-week interval and then begin the next four-week course.

Yarrow Sitz Baths
It's also advisable to take a yarrow sitz bath* once a week. Stay in the bath for twenty minutes, and don't dry yourself off when you get out; put on a robe and get straight into bed. Stay there for an hour so that you work up a good sweat.

Yarrow Tea
Drink two to three cups of yarrow tea* a day, taking care to sip it slowly.

MIGRAINE

Cowslip Tea
If you suffer from severe attacks of migraine, cowslip tea* will bring speedy relief. Drink the tea hot, one sip at a time. You can take up to two cups.

Yarrow Tea
Taking yarrow tea* on a regular basis can eliminate migraine completely. Take one cup of this tea every day, drinking it very hot and taking care to sip it slowly.

MOUTH (infections in)

Mallow Tea
Drink two or three cups of mallow tea* a day, taking care to sip it slowly. It's a good idea to keep your day's supply in a pre-warmed thermos.

Sage Tea
Gargle with sage tea several times a day.

MUCOUS CONGESTION

Nettle Tea
Mucous congestion of the respiratory organs and the stomach can be cleared up with some nettle tea*. Drink one cup a day for several weeks, taking care to sip it slowly.

Sage Tea
Sage also helps to alleviate mucous congestion of the respiratory organs and the stomach. Drink two cups of sage tea* a day, sipping it slowly.

Plantain Tea
Tea made from plantain leaves brings speedy relief in cases of severe mucous congestion of the respiratory organs. Drink two cups of plantain tea* a day, making sure that you sip it slowly.

MUCOUS MEMBRANES (dryness of)

Mallow Tea
Dryness of the mucous membranes in the mouth, throat and nose can be treated with mallow tea*. Gargle and rinse your mouth and throat out with this tea several times a day. To treat dryness of the mucous membranes in the nasal passages you can draw up a little of the cooled tea through your nostrils (do this very gently).

MUSCLES (pulled)

Calendula Tincture Compresses
Calendula tincture* compresses are a very fast-working treatment for pulled muscles. Dilute the tincture with boiled water, moisten a clean cloth with it and apply it to the affected area as a compress.

MUSCLES (swollen)

Swollen muscles — a frequent symptom of rheumatism — can be treated successfully with warm poultices.

Comfrey Root Poultices
Add a tablespoonful of powdered comfrey root and a few drops of vegetable oil to a cupful of hot water and mix thoroughly until smooth. Apply the warm paste to a clean linen cloth and wrap it around the affected muscle.

NAIL INFECTIONS (fungal)

Nettle Footbaths
Stinging nettles are very useful in the treatment of these stubborn and unpleasant fungal infections. Bathe your feet in a nettle footbath* for twenty minutes, without removing the nettles.

Nettle Root Tincture
Nettle root tincture* is also a good remedy. Apply it to the affected nails several times a day.

Nettle Tea
Drink up to four cups of nettle tea* a day, taking care to sip it slowly.

NAIL BED INFECTIONS

Arnica Tincture
Apply arnica tincture* to the affected nails several times a day.

Calendula Ointment
Apply some calendula ointment* to the affected nail.

Chamomile Wash
Pour 1 pt (½l) of hot water into a bowl containing a handful of chamomile flowers and let them steep for half a minute before straining them off. Bathe the affected finger in the warm liquid for twenty minutes and then apply some ointment and a loam poultice.

Garlic Milk
Peel and crush all the cloves from a large head of garlic. Pour 1 pt (½l) of milk into a saucepan, add

the crushed garlic and bring the mixture to the boil. Remove the pan from the heat and bathe your hand in the milk after it has cooled a little.

If there is pus in the finger, you can soak some linseed (flax seed) in water and apply it as a dressing.

After the blister bursts you should bathe the finger in warm chamomile tea and apply St John's wort oil dressings.

Herb Wine
Mix equal quantities of pimpernel, hibiscus, bracken root and elderflowers. Soak ½ oz (15g) of this mixture in 1 pt (½l) of white wine for twelve hours, then heat the infusion up gently and strain it. Allow the wine to cool a little (it should be lukewarm) and then bathe the affected finger in it for two hours. Don't dry the finger afterward; dust it with powdered club moss spores and then bind it gently with a clean cloth or bandage.

Horsetail Footbaths and Wash
Bathe the affected nails carefully with a horsetail wash*.

Soak 4 oz (100g) of horsetail in a bucket of cold water for twelve hours. Then heat up the infusion gently, strain it, and bathe your feet or hands in the warm liquid for twenty minutes.

After taking a footbath or using the horsetail wash you can also wrap the drained horsetail from the infusions in a clean linen cloth and apply it to the affected area as a warm compress.

Mallow Wash
Soak 2 oz (50g) of mallow in cold water for twelve hours. Then heat the infusion up gently, strain it, and bathe the affected hand or foot in the warm liquid for twenty minutes before going to bed. Afterwards, apply calendula ointment* to the infected nails and cover them with a wad of cotton wool moistened with Swedish bitters*, leaving it on overnight.

St John's Wort Oil
Soak a clean cloth or bandage in St John's wort oil* and wrap it around the affected finger.

NAILS (damaged or brittle)

You can treat brittle, broken or injured nails with fresh crowfoot juice or onion juice.

Cut open the thick stems of a fresh crowfoot plant and apply the juice that it exudes directly to your nails. This should be repeated every day.

Cut an onion in half and rub your nails with the cut surface several times a day.

Walnut Leaf Tea
Suppurating, infected fingernails and toenails can be treated by bathing them in walnut leaf tea* several times a day.

NAUSEA

Hawthorn Tea
Drink two cups of hawthorn tea* in the course of the day, taking care to sip it slowly.

Hawthorn Tincture
Take between four and ten drops of hawthorn tincture* every day.

Swedish Bitters
According to Dr. Samst's old manuscript, Swedish bitters* are also effective in treating giddiness and nausea. Take up to three teaspoons of the bitters a day, dissolved in a little of one of the herbs teas described here.

Yarrow Tea
Drink one or two cups of yarrow tea* during the day, taking care to sip it slowly.

NECK (stiff)

Comfrey Root Poultices
Hot comfrey root poultices bring rapid relief from a stiff neck. Add a tablespoon of powdered comfrey and a few drops of vegetable oil to a cup of hot water and mix them thoroughly until the consistency is smooth. Apply the warm paste to a clean linen cloth and wrap the cloth around your neck, binding it gently into place with a warm cloth.

NERVOUSNESS

Speedwell Tea
Stress at home or at work is often the cause of increased nervousness. Speedwell is a very soothing plant and brings rapid relief. Drink one cup of speedwell tea* before going to bed at night, taking care to sip it slowly.

St John's Wort Tea
Drink two to three cups of St John's wort tea* a day, taking care to sip it slowly.

NIGHT SWEATS

Herbal Mixture
Mix ¾ oz (20g) of lady's mantle with ¾ oz (20g) of lavender, ¾ oz (20g) of sage and ¾ oz (20g) of horsetail. Drink one cup of tea brewed from this mixture every day before breakfast, taking care to sip it slowly. Use one heaping teaspoonful of the mixture for each cup of tea. Pour on hot water and let the herbs steep for thirty seconds before straining them off.

Sage Tea
Drink two cups of sage tea* a day, one before breakfast and one before going to bed. Take care to sip it slowly.

NIPPLES (inflammation of)

Swedish Bitters
Apply Swedish bitters* to your nipples with cotton wool several times a day, continuing the treatment until the soreness has gone.

NOSEBLEEDS

Horsetail Compresses
Cold compresses made with horsetail tea* can help to stem severe, long-lasting nosebleeds. Let the tea cool completely and then soak a cloth in it and lay it over your nose.

Mistletoe Tea
Sniff a little cool mistletoe tea* very gently into your nostrils — this helps to stem the bleeding.

Shepherd's Purse Tea
Chronic nosebleeds can be cured with the help of shepherd's purse tea*.

Yarrow Tea
Drink a cup of yarrow tea* very slowly, one sip at a time.

OBESITY

Hawthorn Tea
Drink at least four cups of hawthorn tea* a day, taking care to sip it slowly.

Hawthorn Tincture
Take between four and ten drops of hawthorn tincture* a day.

Lady's Mantle Tea
At higher altitudes, up to around 4,000 ft (1300m), one finds a variety of lady's mantle known as alpine lady's mantle. The undersides of the leaves are silvery, making it easy to identify. Tea made from these leaves can be helpful in cases of obesity and overweight.

Use one heaping teaspoonful of the silvery leaves, finely chopped, for each cup of tea. Pour on hot water and let the leaves steep for thirty seconds before straining them off. Drink two to three cups of this tea a day, taking care to sip it slowly.

Wild Chicory Tea
Drink two cups of wild chicory tea* a day, taking care to sip it slowly.

OPERATION SCARS

Calendula Ointment
Applying calendula ointment* to operation scars every day helps them to heal more quickly.

OVEREXCITEMENT

Thyme baths
If you become nervous and overexcited too easily, a thyme bath* once or twice a week can work wonders. It's important that your heart should not be below the water level. Stay in the bath for twenty minutes and don't dry yourself off when you get out; put on a robe and get straight into bed. Stay there for an hour so that you work up a good sweat.

OVEREXERTION

Comfrey Root Poultices
Warm poultices made with a paste of powdered comfrey root are very helpful in cases of physical overexertion.

Add a tablespoon of powdered comfrey root and a few drops of vegetable oil to a cup of hot water and mix them well until the consistency is smooth. Apply the hot paste to a clean linen cloth, wrap it around the affected area while it is still hot and bind it into place with a second cloth to keep in the heat.

Speedwell Tea

The nervous tension that is often caused by mental overexertion can be alleviated with the help of speedwell tea.* Drink one cup in the evening before going to sleep, taking care to sip it slowly.

St John's Wort Tea

St John's wort tea* is another good remedy for physical overexertion. Drink two to three cups every day, taking care to sip it slowly.

OVERWEIGHT

Maize Tassel Tea

Maize tassel tea* is a natural, effective and rapid way of dealing with excess weight. Drink up to four cups a day, taking care to sip it slowly.

Wild Chicory Tea

Drink one cup of wild chicory tea* every day before breakfast, taking care to sip it slowly.

PAINS

Swedish bitters

Swedish bitters* are very effective for relieving all sorts of pains, whatever the site of the discomfort. Depending on the severity of the pain, take between a teaspoonful and a tablespoonful of Swedish bitters three times a day, dissolved in a little water or herb tea. You can also apply diluted Swedish bitters externally, either by rubbing it into the skin directly or by moistening a wad of cotton wool with it and applying it as a compress, binding it into place with a clean linen cloth or a bandage. It's a good idea to apply calendula ointment* to the affected area first, however, so that the alcohol in the Swedish bitters doesn't draw the natural oils out of your skin.

PALLOR

Lady's Mantle Tea

Drink two or three cups of lady's mantle tea* a day, taking care to sip it slowly.

Plantain Tea

Plantain has blood-purifying properties, and also helps to clean out the stomach and the lungs, so it can be recommended for anyone who suffers from pallor. Drink one or two cups of plantain tea* a day, sipping it slowly.

PERIODS (irregular)

Lady's Mantle and Yarrow Tea

This tea is very useful for dealing with period problems during puberty — missed periods and irregular periods, for instance.

Mix equal quantities of lady's mantle and yarrow. Use one heaping teaspoonful of the mixture for each cup of tea. Pour on hot water and let the herbs steep for thirty seconds before straining them off. Drink two cups of this tea every day for quite a while, taking care to sip it slowly.

Shepherd's Purse Tea

Both shepherd's purse tea* and St John's wort tea (see above) are excellent for normalizing periods during puberty. In the week before your period is due to start, drink two cups of this tea every day. Take care to drink the tea slowly, one sip at a time.

St John's Wort Tea

Drink two cups of St John's wort tea* a day for quite a while.

PHARYNGITIS

Coltsfoot Tea

Drink two or three cups of coltsfoot tea* a day, sweetened with a little honey. Take care to sip it slowly.

PRURITUS SENILIS

Speedwell Tea

Drink two cups of speedwell tea* a day, sipping it slowly.

Yarrow Tea

Drink two or three cups of yarrow tea* a day, taking care to sip it slowly.

PSORIASIS

This terrible disease is commonly regarded as incurable, but in my experience it really is possible to treat it with the help of medicinal herbs from God's garden.

Diet

Since this so-called incurable disease is caused by a dysfunction of the liver, the first thing to do is to start eating a strict liver diet and to adhere to it religiously.

The combination of a liver diet and the herbal treatments described below can also be used to treat neurodermatitis.

Baths

Take three herbal baths a week, with infusions made from either cranesbill or a mixture of equal parts of mallow and horsetail.

Take 8 oz (200g) of the herbs for each bath and soak them in 1 gal (5l) of cold water for twelve hours. Then heat up the infusion gently and strain the liquid into your bathwater. It's important that your heart should not be below the water level. Stay in the bath for twenty minutes, and don't dry yourself off when you get out; put on a dressing gown and get straight into bed, staying there for an hour so that you work up a good sweat.

Embrocations

Apply some pure lard to the skin twice a day. If the psoriasis has broken open or become en-crusted, you should mix the lard with fresh celandine juice to make an ointment before applying it. To make the juice wash some freshly-picked celandine and run it through a juice extractor. Add ¼ oz (5g) of celandine juice to 12½ oz (50g) of lard and blend them well. This ointment must be kept in the refrigerator. If you wish you can use fresh mallow juice instead of celandine juice.

Herbal Mixture

Mix 2½ oz (50g) of stinging nettles, 1½ oz (30g) of speedwell, ½ oz (10g) of oak bark, 1 oz (20g) of fumaria, 1½ oz (30g) of calendula, 1 oz (20g) of yarrow, 1½ oz (30g) of celandine, 1 oz (20g) of walnut shells, 1½ oz (30g) of willow bark and 2 oz (40g) of meadowsweet.

Drink six to eight cups of tea brewed from this mixture in the course of the day. Use one heaping teaspoonful of the mixture for each cup of tea. Pour on hot water and let the herbs steep for thirty seconds before straining them off. Drink the tea slowly, one sip at a time. Use fresh herbs if at all possible, as they are more potent than the dried ones.

RASHES AND SKIN ERUPTIONS

Chamomile Compresses

Rashes and skin eruptions can be treated successfully by applying chamomile compresses and bathing the affected area with a chamomile wash.

Pour ½ pt (¼l) of boiling milk into a bowl containing a heaping teaspoonful of chamomile, and let it steep for half a minute before straining it. Let the milk cool until it is hand-hot, then soak a clean linen cloth in it and apply the cloth directly to the affected area.

Chamomile Wash

Bathe the affected areas with a chamomile wash* as soon as it is cool enough to be bearable.

Dandelion Stems

Eat ten raw, freshly-picked dandelion stems every day, washing them carefully beforehand and chewing them very thoroughly. Don't cut off the flowers until after you have washed the plants. This treatment should be continued for as long as the dandelions are in flower.

Plantain Tea

Drink two cups of plantain* tea a day, taking care to sip it slowly.

Swedish Bitters

Apply some Swedish bitters* to the affected areas several times a day with a wad of cotton wool.

Walnut Leaf Wash

Even the most stubborn rashes and pus-filled eruptions can be healed by bathing the affected area with a walnut leaf wash*.

RESTLESSNESS

Yarrow Sitz Baths
It's a good idea to complement the effects of yarrow tea with a yarrow sitz bath*, as this brings even more rapid relief. The water should be just deep enough to cover your kidneys. Stay in the bath for twenty minutes and don't dry yourself off when you get out; put on a robe and get straight into bed. Stay there for an hour so that you work up a good sweat.

Yarrow Tea
Yarrow has soothing properties which can help to alleviate restlessness. Drink two to three cups of yarrow tea* a day, taking care to sip it slowly.

RHEUMATISM

Agrimony Tea
Drink two cups of agrimony tea* a day, taking care to sip it slowly.

Chamomile oil
Chamomile oil* is a good treatment for rheumatism. Apply it to the affected areas regularly, massaging it in gently.

Club Moss Tea
Drink one cup of club moss tea* a day before breakfast, taking care to sip it slowly.

Comfrey Baths
An infusion of comfrey leaves makes an excellent bath essence for treating rheumatism. Soak 1 lb (500g) of comfrey leaves in 1 gal (5l) of cold water for twelve hours, then heat up the infusion gently and strain it into your bathwater. It is important that your heart should be above the water level. Stay in the bath for twenty minutes and don't dry yourself off when you get out; put on a robe and get straight into bed. Stay there for an hour so that you work up a good sweat.

Comfrey Root Tincture
Rub the affected joints with comfrey root tincture* every day — you will find that this brings speedy relief.

Cowslip Tea
Drink one or two cups of cowslip tea* a day, taking care to sip it slowly.

Dandelion Stems
Eat ten raw, freshly-picked dandelion stems every day, washing them carefully beforehand and chewing them very thoroughly. Don't cut off the flowers until after you have washed the plants. This treatment is only possible in the spring, as the dandelions must be picked while they are in flower.

Horsetail Tea
Drink one cup of horsetail tea* a day, taking care to sip it slowly.

This tea is a good preventive remedy, providing effective protection against gout, rheumatism and neuralgia, as long as you start taking it early enough.

Maize Tassel Tea
Drink one or two cups of maize tassel tea* a day, taking care to sip it slowly.

Meadowsweet Tea
Drink two to three cups of meadowsweet tea* a day, taking care to sip it slowly.

Nettle Baths
Nettle baths* are another effective remedy for gout and rheumatism. It's important that your heart should be above the water level. Stay in the bath for twenty minutes and don't dry yourself off when you get out; put on a robe and get straight into bed. Stay there for an hour so that you work up a good sweat.

Speedwell Tincture
Speedwell tincture* is a good external remedy for rheumatism. Massage a little of this tincture into the affected areas every day.

As an additional measure, you can take speedwell tincture internally. Take fifteen drops three times a day, dissolved in a little water or herb tea.

St John's Wort Oil
St John's wort oil* is of proven value in the treatment of rheumatism. Rub into the affected joint.

Swedish Bitters
Take one teaspoonful of Swedish bitters* three times a day, dissolved in a little nettle tea* or horsetail tea*.

As an additional measure, you can apply Swedish bitters externally. Moisten a wad of cotton wool with some bitters and lay it on the affected area as a compress. It's a good idea to apply some calendula ointment* beforehand so that the alcohol in the bitters doesn't draw the natural oils out of your skin.

Thyme Oil
Thyme oil* is yet another effective external remedy for rheumatism. Apply the oil directly to the affected joints.

Yarrow Tea
Take up to four cups of yarrow tea* a day, drinking it as hot as you can bear it and taking care to sip it slowly.

RINGWORM

Walnut Leaf Wash
A walnut leaf wash* brings rapid relief. Rinse the affected areas with the liquid, massaging it in well.

SCABIES

Calendula Juice
Run the stems of some freshly-picked calendula plants through a juice extractor and apply the juice directly to the affected areas.

Knotgrass Wash
Pour 1 pt (½ l) of hot water into a bowl containing two generous handfuls of knotgrass. Let the knotgrass steep for thirty seconds before straining it off. Bathe the affected areas with the liquid.

Walnut Leaf Wash
Walnut leaf wash* brings speedy relief from scabies. Bathe the affected areas with the liquid.

SCALDS

> ### Home Remedy
> *An alternative first-aid remedy is to apply the white of an egg to a clean linen cloth and to wrap it around the scald. Again, go to the doctor as soon as possible after administering first-aid!*

St John's Wort Oil
It is very important to use *linseed* oil for making St John's wort oil* when it is to be used for treating scalds and burns. Apply the oil directly to the scald as a first-aid measure and then go to the doctor without delay.

SCARS

Calendula Ointment
Operation wounds heal more quickly and leave less of a scar if you apply calendula ointment* to them regularly.

You can also use the ointment in dressings. Apply a generous quantity to a clean linen cloth and wrap it around the wound, binding it into place with another cloth to keep the warmth in. This dressing should be changed once a day. Don't throw the drained herbs and any other residue away after you make the ointment — they can be used to make an excellent warm compress.

Swedish Bitters
In Dr. Samst's old manuscript, in which the recipe for these bitters was found, it is claimed that scars disappear almost completely after about forty applications of Swedish bitters*. Dab the bitters directly onto the scar with a little cotton wool.

SINUSITIS

Chamomile tea
Drink three cups of chamomile tea* in the course of the day, taking care to sip it slowly.

SINUSITIS (frontal)

Swedish Bitters Compresses
Swedish bitters* compresses are a good remedy for both normal and suppurative sinusitis. Apply some calendula ointment* to your forehead before you put the compress on in order to prevent the alcohol in the bitters from drawing the natural oils out of your skin. Then moisten a wad of cotton wool with Swedish bitters and lay it over the affected area, covering it with a layer of dry cotton wool and a layer of plastic film to keep the warmth in, and bind it all gently into place with a warm cloth. Apply the compress in the evening before going to sleep and leave it on all night.

SKIN CARE (facial)

Bedstraw Tea
Applied externally, bedstraw tea* can help to firm and tighten your skin, smoothing out wrinkles. Bathe your face with the tea several times a day.

St John's Wort Oil
St John's wort oil* can help to smooth coarse skin. If you massage your face with this oil every day, coarse skin will soon become soft and supple.

SKIN RASHES

Chamomile wash
Bathe your face with a chamomile wash* every day.

Deadnettle Tea
Drink one cup of deadnettle tea every morning, taking care to sip it slowly.

Horsetail Wash
Bathe your face and the other affected areas with a horsetail wash* every day. Alternatively, you can soak a clean linen cloth in the warm horsetail wash and wrap it around the affected area.

Sorrel Tea
Drink two cups of sorrel tea* a day, taking care to sip it slowly.

SLEEPWALKING

St John's Wort Sitz Baths
In addition to the tea it's also advisable to take one St John's wort sitz bath* and six St John's wort footbaths every week.

The sitz bath water should be just deep enough to cover your kidneys. Stay in the bath for twenty minutes, and don't dry yourself off when you get out; put on a robe and get straight into bed. Stay there for an hour so that you work up a good sweat.

You only need half as much St John's wort for the daily footbaths. Prepare the infusion using the standard method for the St John's wort sitz bath*.

St John's Wort Tea
Drink two cups of St John's wort tea* a day, taking care to sip it slowly.

SMOKER'S COMPLAINTS

Coltsfoot Juice
Excessive smoking leads to shortness of breath and a nasty, chronic cough. If you suffer from these complaints, a treatment with coltsfoot juice can work wonders. (As with all regenerative cures, the spring is the best time for this.) Take between two and three teaspoons of coltsfoot leaf juice a day, dissolved in a cup of meat broth or hot milk. Always use fresh coltsfoot leaves and make the juice fresh, just before you drink it.

SMOKING

Calamus Roots
If you're trying to stop smoking and your willpower just isn't up to it, you will find that the roots of the calamus can be very helpful. Instead of lighting a cigarette, take a little dried, finely-chopped calamus root and chew it very slowly and carefully, spitting out the woody remains when all the juice is gone. The spicy, bitter juice of the roots helps to relieve withdrawal symptoms, and if you do weaken and light up a cigarette you'll find that it tastes really revolting!

SPOTS AND PIMPLES (facial)

Bedstraw Ointment
Bedstraw oitment is another excellent remedy for spots and pimples.

Melt 1 lb (500g) of pure lard in a saucepan and add four generous handfuls of bedstraw. Proceed according to the standard recipe for ointment.*

Bedstraw Wash
Bathe the affected area several times a day with a bedstraw wash*.

Calendula Juice
Run some fresh calendula stems through a juice extractor and apply the juice to the spots several times a day.

Cedar Tincture
Apply cedar tincture* to the spots several times a day.

Houseleek Sap

Take some fresh houseleek leaves, wash them, cut them into long thin strips and apply the sap that they exude to the affected areas.

SPRAINS

Arnica Tincture

Sprains can be treated by massaging the affected area with arnica tincture*. Compresses containing the petals used to make the arnica tincture are also an effective remedy.

Butterbur Leaf Dressings

Wash some freshly-picked butterbur leaves, crush them to a pulp on a wooden chopping board using a rolling pin and spread the pulp on the sprin.

Thyme Oil

Sprains can also be treated by massaging them gently with thyme oil*. Apply the thyme oil to the sprain several times a day.

STITCH

Bedstraw Tea

Bedstraw tea* brings speedy relief from a stitch. Drink two to three cups a day, taking care to sip it slowly.

STOMACH (disorders of)

Mallow Tea

Drink two cups of mallow tea* in the course of the day, taking care to sip it slowly. It's a good idea to keep your day's supply in a pre-warmed thermos.

Swedish Bitters

Swedish bitters* are also a good remedy for stomach disorders. Take three teaspoonfuls a day in a little water or herb tea.

STOMACH (heaviness and feelings of pressure in)

Yarrow Tea

Drink two cups of yarrow tea* a day (one in the morning and one in the evening), taking care to sip it slowly.

STOMACH (wind in)

Calamus Root Tea

Drink one mouthful of calamus root tea* before and after each meal, i.e., a total of six mouthfuls a day. This is equivalent to one cup, and it is important not to drink more than this quantity in the course of the day. It's a good idea to keep your day's supply in a pre-warmed thermos.

STOMACH-ACHES

Calamus Root Tea

Calamus root tea* is a good treatment for adults who have stomach-ache. Drink one mouthful before and after each meal. (Don't drink more than six mouthfuls a day — this is equivalent to one cup.) It's best to keep the tea in a pre-warmed thermos, as it cools off very quickly.

Chamomile Tea

The soothing, healing properties of chamomile are of equal value for both adults and children. Take up to three cups of chamomile tea* a day, depending on the severity of the stomach-ache. Drink the tea slowly, one sip at a time.

St John's Wort Oil

For small children and babies, an excellent way of treating stomach-ache is to apply St John's wort oil* externally, massaging it gently into the skin over their tummies.

STOMACH CRAMPS

Calendula Tea

Drink two cups of calendula tea* a day (one in the morning and one in the evening), taking care to sip it slowly.

Club Moss Compresses

Fill a pillowcase with 4 to 8 oz (100-200g) of club moss and apply it to your stomach as a compress.

Horsetail Compresses

Hot horsetail compresses bring rapid relief from painful stomach cramps. Put two generous handfuls of horsetail in a sieve and heat it up over boiling water. Don't let the horsetail come into contact with the water! Then wrap the horsetail in a clean linen cloth and apply it to the affected area, leaving it in place for several hours. If you wish you can also apply the compress in the evening and leave it on overnight. It's important to wear warm clothes over the compress to keep the heat in, otherwise the healing horsetail vapors will be wasted.

Nettle Tea
Drink up to three cups of nettle tea* a day, taking care to sip it slowly.

Swedish Bitters
As soon as you feel an attack of stomach cramps coming on, it's a good idea to take a tablespoonful of Swedish bitters*, dissolving it in a little water or herb tea. You can take up to three tablespoons of the bitters a day, depending on the severity of the cramps.

Thyme Compresses
A thyme compress can also bring relief from stomach cramps. Fill a small pillowcase or cushion cover loosely with dried thyme blossoms and stems, and apply it to the affected area.

Thyme Tea
Drink two cups of thyme tea* in the course of the day, taking care to sip it slowly.

Yarrow Tea
Drink one cup of yarrow tea* in the morning and another in the evening, taking care to sip it slowly.

STOMATITIS (sore mouth)

Agrimony Tea
Gargle with agrimony tea* several times a day.

Horsetail Tea
Gargle with horsetail tea* several times a day.

Mallow Tea
Drink two or three cups of mallow tea* a day, taking care to sip it slowly. It's a good idea to keep your day's supply in a pre-warmed thermos.

Sage Tea
Gargle with sage tea* several times a day.

Walnut Leaf Tea
Rinsing out your mouth several times a day with walnut leaf tea helps to alleviate ulcerative stomatitis.

SUNBURN

Club Moss Spores
Dust the burned skin very gently with powdered club moss spores. This powder draws the heat and moisture out of the burns.

St John's Wort Oil
For treating sunburn and all other types of burns, St John's wort oil* must be made with *linseed* oil. Apply the oil to the sunburned skin several times a day.

TEAR GLANDS (lacrimal glands)

Herbal Mixture
Compresses made from an infusion of the following herbal mixture are an excellent remedy for chronically watering eyes.

Mix ½ oz (10g) of eyebright, ½ oz (10g) of valerian, ¾ oz (15g) of blessed thistle root, ½ oz (10g) of lilac blossoms, ¾ oz (15g) of lady's mantle, 1 oz (20g) of chamomile and ½ oz (10g) of ruewort.

Soak ¾ oz (15g) of this mixture in 1 pt (½l) of water for twelve hours, then heat up the infusion gently and strain it. Soak a clean cloth in the warm liquid and apply it directly to your eyes (keep your eyes closed). Renew the compress after half an hour. After another thirty minutes, remove the compress, replace it with a warm, dry cloth or towel, and rest quietly for a while.

Mallow Tea
In cases where the flow of lacrimal fluid stops and the eyes become almost completely dry, treatment with mallow tea* used as an eyewash and in compresses is often quite effective.

To bathe your eyes with this tea it's best to use an eyebath, which you can obtain at any chemist's. Alternatively, you can soak a clean cloth in the tea and apply it to your closed eyes as a compress.

Yarrow Tea
Yarrow tea* can be very helpful in treating chronically watering eyes. Drink two or three cups of this tea a day, taking care to sip it slowly.

TEETH (extracted)

Lady's Mantle Tea

After having a tooth extracted, gargle and rinse out your mouth with cooled lady's mantle tea* several times a day.

TEETH (loose)

Herbal Mixture

Mix equal quantities of oak bark, lady's mantle, sage and knotgrass. Soak two heaping teaspoons of this mixture in 1 pt (½l) of water for twelve hours, and then heat up the infusion gently and strain it. Rinse your mouth out with this tea several times a day. It's a good idea to keep your day's supply in a pre-warmed thermos. In addition to using this tea as a mouthwash, you should massage it gently into your gums with a soft toothbrush.

Sage Tea

Gargle with sage tea* several times a day. As an additional measure, soak a wad of cotton wool in sage tea and place it against the loose tooth.

THROAT INFECTIONS

Agrimony Tea

Gargle with agrimony tea* twice a day, once in the morning and once in the evening.

Bedstraw Tea

Gargle with bedstraw tea* several times a day.

Sage Tea

Gargle with sage tea* twice a day; once in the morning and once in the evening.

You can also use the tea to make compresses. Moisten a wad of cotton wool with the tea and apply it to your throat, binding it gently into place with a cloth or bandage.

Swedish Bitters

Take three teaspoons of Swedish bitters* a day, dissolving each teaspoonful in half a cup of herb tea. Divide each dose into two portions, drinking one half an hour before each meal and one half an hour afterward.

THROAT (sore)

Agrimony Tea

Gargle with agrimony tea* twice a day.

Sage Tea

Gargle with sage tea* twice a day, once in the morning and once in the evening.

It's a good idea to apply a sage tea compress as well. Soak a large wad of cotton wool in the tea, wring it out and apply it to your throat, binding it gently into place with a bandage or a clean cloth.

Walnut Leaf Tea

Gargle with walnut leaf tea* twice a day, once in the morning and once in the evening.

TIREDNESS

Chamomile oil

Feelings of physical tiredness and heaviness can be treated with chamomile oil*. Gently massage your entire body with the oil before going to bed at night.

Nettle Tea

Drink up to four cups of nettle tea* a day, taking care to sip it slowly.

Peppermint Tea

Use one heaping teaspoonful of peppermint for each cup of tea. Pour on hot water and let the herbs steep for thirty seconds before straining them off. Drink up to three cups of this tea a day, taking care to sip it slowly.

TONGUE (blisters on)

Swedish Bitters

Small blisters on the tongue, which are often caused by eating one's food too hot, are best treated with Swedish bitters*.

Take one tablespoonful of the bitters three times a day, diluting it in a little water or herb tea and slooshing it around your mouth for a while before swallowing it.

TONGUE (furred)

Wormwood Tea

Wormwood tea is a very old remedy for a furred tongue. You should be very careful with wormwood, however, as it is nowhere near as harmless as is commonly believed — don't use more than half a teaspoonful to make one cup of tea. If you like, you can use a hot herb tea instead of plain water when making wormwood tea.

TONGUE
(swollen or scalded)

Bedstraw Tea
Pains and swelling of the tongue, or minor scalds caused by eating one's food too hot, can be treated with tea made from fresh bedstraw. You will need enough freshly-picked, finely-chopped bedstraw to make between six and eight cups of tea a day. Keep your day's supply in a thermos.

Rinse your mouth out with bedstraw tea* several times a day, swallowing down a mouthful every time you do so. Continue the treatment for several days, until the symptoms have disappeared.

TONSILLITIS

Mallow Tea
Mallow is rich in mucin and brings speedy relief from tonsillitis. Drink two to three cups of mallow tea* a day, taking care to sip it slowly. It's a good idea to keep your day's supply in a pre-warmed thermos.

Sage Compresses
Pour 1 pt (½l) of water into a bowl containing two teaspoonfuls of sage and let it steep for thirty seconds before straining it. Soak a clean linen cloth in the liquid and wrap it around your throat. It's very important to keep the heat in — it's best to wrap a dry towel or a warm cloth over the wet compress. Change the compress several times a day. It's also a good idea to gargle thoroughly with the sage infusion several times a day.

St John's Wort and Horsetail Tea
A herb tea made from equal measures of St John's wort and horsetail makes a good gargle for tonsillitis. Use one heaping teaspoonful of this mixture for each cup of tea. Pour on hot water and let the herbs steep for thirty seconds before straining them off. Gargle with this tea several times a day.

TOOTHACHE

Chamomile Tea
Drink up to three cups of chamomile tea* a day, taking care to sip it slowly. It's also a good idea to rinse your mouth out with it several times a day.

Swedish Bitters
Take a tablespoonful of Swedish bitters* diluted with a little water or herb tea and sloosh it around your mouth for a while before swallowing it. It also helps to soak a wad of cotton wool with Swedish bitters and to place it against the aching tooth.

UNDERWEIGHT

Calamus Root Baths
In addition to drinking calamus root tea it's also advisable to take an occasional calamus root bath*. It's important that your heart should be above the water level. Stay in the bath for twenty minutes, and don't dry yourself off when you get out; put on a robe and get straight into bed. Stay there for an hour so that you work up a good sweat.

Calamus Root Tea
If you don't seem to be able to put on weight, even though you eat plenty of good nourishing food, you may very well have a metabolic disorder, which is a frequent cause of underweight. In cases like this calamus root tea* can help to improve the situation.

Drink one mouthful of this tea before and after each meal, i.e., a total of six mouthfuls a day. This is equivalent to one cup, and it is important not to drink more than this quantity in the course of the day. It's a good idea to keep your day's supply in a pre-warmed thermos.

VARICOSE VEINS

Agrimony Ointment
Both this ointment and calendula ointment bring speedy relief from varicose veins. Gently massage some of the ointment into the whole affected area every day.

Melt 8 oz (250g) of pure lard in a saucepan and add two generous handfuls of finely-chopped agrimony leaves, flowers and stems. Proceed according to the standard recipe for ointment*.

Calendula Ointment
Calendula ointment is another very effective and fast-acting remedy for varicose veins.

Melt 8 oz (250g) of pure lard in a saucepan and add two generous handfuls of calendula leaves, stems and flowers. Proceed according to the standard recipe for calendula ointment*.

You can also use the calendula ointment in leg compresses. Apply a generous amount of the ointment to your legs (if you've just made the ointment you can also use the strained calendula itself) and cover it with a clean bandage or linen cloth. Change the compress every day.

Comfrey Sitz Baths

Soak 8 oz (200g) of fresh or dried comfrey leaves in 8 pt (5l) of cold water for twelve hours, then heat the infusion up gently and strain it into your bathwater. The water should be just deep enough to cover your kidneys. Stay in the bath for twenty minutes, and don't dry yourself off when you get out; put on a robe and get straight into bed. Stay there for an hour so that you work up a good sweat.

Deadnettle Compresses

Deadnettle compresses are another excellent way of treating painful varicose veins.

Pour 1 pt (½l) of hot water into a bowl containing three heaping teaspoonfuls of deadnettles and let them steep for thirty seconds. Soak some clean linen cloths in the liquid, wring them out gently and wrap them around your legs.

VOMITING

Swedish Bitters

Take two or three tablespoonfuls of Swedish bitters* a day, dissolving each tablespoonful in half a cup of herb tea. Divide each of these doses into two portions, taking one of them half an hour before eating and the other half an hour afterwards.

Swedish Bitters Compresses

Apply some calendula ointment* before putting on the compress to prevent the alcohol in the Swedish bitters* from drawing the natural oils out of your skin. Moisten a large wad of cotton wool with Swedish bitters and place it over your stomach, binding it into place with a bandage or a linen cloth. You can leave the compress on for between two and four hours.

WARTS

Arnica Tincture

Soak a small wad of cotton wool with arnica tincture* and press it firmly against the wart for a few moments.

Calendula Juice

Direct applications of fresh calendula juice can heal both warts and scabies. Wash some fresh calendula leaves, blossoms and stems and run them through a juice extractor without drying them off first.

Celandine Juice

Fresh celandine juice is another effective remedy. Wash some freshly picked celandine leaves, blossoms and stems and run them through a juice extractor without drying them off first. Apply the fresh juice directly to the warts.

Swedish Bitters

Apply a little Swedish bitters* to the warts several times a day when a small wad of cotton wool, continuing until they disappear.

WASP STINGS

See Insect Bites.

WEAKNESS (general)

Horsetail Tea

Drink at least one cup of horsetail tea* every day, taking care to sip it slowly.

Mistletoe Tea

Drink up to three cups of mistletoe tea* a day, taking care to sip it slowly. It's a good idea to keep your day's supply in a pre-warmed thermos.

WORMS

Calendula Tea

Drink one cup of calendula tea* a day, taking care to sip it slowly.

Pumpkin Seeds

Pumpkin seeds are an old household remedy for threadworms. Children should eat ten to fifteen shelled pumpkin seeds every day; adults, twenty to thirty. When you are shelling the seeds try to leave the fine inner skin beneath the shell intact, as it is very important to eat this with the seeds. Chew them very thoroughly, and take half a teaspoonful of castor oil one hour later.

More pumpkin seeds need to be eaten if tapeworms are the problem. Keep to a healthy diet, and take between twenty and twenty-five shelled pumpkin seeds four times a day. Take half a teaspoonful of castor oil one hour after each dose of seeds. You can repeat this treatment as often as necessary without any danger of side-effects.

Roundworms can be eliminated if you eat raw carrots and beetroot. Chew them well and wash them down with raw sauerkraut juice. Another good way of getting rid of roundworms quickly is to boil some garlic, horseradish and onions in milk and to drink it as hot as possible but slowly — one little sip at a time.

Ramsons (Broad-leaved Garlic)

Ramson's healing properties include the ability to eliminate intestinal worms. The fresh leaves can be collected in the spring and should be eaten raw. Wash the leaves, chop them up finely, and sprinkle them on your food as you would fresh parsley. Spinach tastes lovely if you cook it together with a few ramsons leaves, and they also make an excellent addition to salads.

Ramsons (Broad-leaved Garlic) Tincture

Take between ten and fifteen drops of ramsons tincture* four times a day, dissolved in a little water.

Sorrel Tea

Drink two cups of sorrel tea* a day, sipping it slowly.

Swedish Bitters

Take three teaspoons of Swedish bitters* a day, dissolving each teaspoonful in half a cup of one of the herb teas described above. Divide each of these three doses into two portions, taking one of them before eating and the other one afterwards.

Moisten a small cloth with Swedish bitters and dab it on your navel, applying a little calendula ointment* first.

4. Faith Can Move Mountains

The illnesses in the following list can only be diagnosed by a doctor, and diagnoses should not be attempted by anyone else. Nowadays there are fewer conflicts between the approach of orthodox medicine and your faith in the healing power of the herbs that can be found in God's garden. A good doctor will never tell you not to use medicinal herbs, for he will be aware of the fact that herbal remedies always help, they never hinder!

The health and well-being of the patient is more important than anything else, and it is only natural that we should expect our doctors to understand this. In addition to this it is important to remember that there is no law that forces you to be a passive bystander simply because you are ill: you have every right to take an active part in your own treatment.

As I see it, a good doctor ought to be delighted when his patients are willing to take their share of the responsibility for their own recovery, for in such cases all the problems involved and the possible ways of solving them can be discussed openly. And remember, it is *always* up to you to decide whether your doctor may do something or not! This becomes most apparent in the case of surgical operations, where one usually has to sign a form giving the surgeon permission to operate, but in actual fact every doctor needs your tacit consent before he is allowed to do anything, however minor it may seem.

Please, don't misunderstand me. I am not attempting to cause trouble, I am simply trying to rectify what I regard as a very unfortunate situation. So many of my readers have written to tell me that they use medicinal herbs secretly because they are afraid of what their doctors would say if they knew. For instance, in one letter I received a little while ago a man confided in me that he hadn't told his doctors anything about the fact that he was treating himself with medicinal herbs. "Why should I?" he wrote. "Let them go on believing that it was their tinkering which made me get better. Even if I did tell them, they'd never believe that it was your herbs that were responsible for my recovery, and not their treatment!"

But, I ask myself, why is it that people feel that they can't confide in their doctors? After all, they *are* doctors — and any doctor's primary concern must surely be the health and well-being of his patients, for that is his job and his vocation!

Whatever their reasons, I am sure that there will be many people who will criticize me when they see that I claim that medicinal herbs can even be of help in the treatment of illnesses such as multiple sclerosis or psoriasis. They will say that it is irresponsible of me to raise false hopes in people whose cases the doctors have given up as hopeless.

Such attacks do not impress me in the least. My own faith and my experience have taught me that improvement and healing are possible even in the most desperate cases. I have no idea *why* medicinal herbs work, nor do I know with certainty whether faith is more important than the herb. I only know one thing for sure, and that is that no matter whether we are sick or healthy we are all completely lost without firm faith in God's grace and omnipotence.

For example, if a cancer patient who has been told that nothing can be done for him simply accepts his fate passively, it is unlikely that he will live very long. Only if he refuses to allow himself to be overcome by feelings of hopelessness does he have a chance of conquering his illness. The first step on the way to healing is to pluck up the courage to take our destiny into our own hands again.

The importance of this positive, responsible attitude toward one's own health has been confirmed by a study conducted by the American neurophysiologist, Dr. Herbert Spector, in which he observed a number of breast cancer patients over a period of ten years. He found that the women could be divided into two groups on the basis of their attitude and their reaction to their illness. One group fought the disease actively, refusing to believe that they were at the mercy of their fate, whereas the other group became passive and resigned, abandoning their will to live. At the end of the ten years eighty per cent of the women in the active group were still alive, and ninety per cent of the women in the passive group had died.

Faith can move mountains. This is something we have all heard again and again, but very few of us really understand just how much comfort, hope and courage these four simple words can give. And hand in hand with the medicinal herbs from God's garden, faith can help all of us to find new courage and overcome what may seem to be hopeless and desperate situations.

ADENOIDS

St John's Wort and Horsetail Tea
Mix equal quantities of St John's wort and horsetail. Use one heaping teaspoonful of this mixture for each cup of tea. Pour on hot water and let the herbs steep for thirty seconds before straining them off. Gargle with this tea several times a day.

ANEMIA

Agrimony Tea
Drink up to two cups of agrimony tea* a day, taking care to sip them slowly.

Lady's Mantle Tea
Drink up to three cups of lady's mantle tea* in the course of the day, taking care to sip it slowly.

Nettle Tea
The stinging nettle helps to stimulate the production of fresh blood cells, which makes it indispensable in dealing with anemia. Drink up to four cups of nettle tea* a day, taking care to sip it slowly.

Swedish Bitters
Take one tablespoonful of Swedish bitters* every day, dissolving it in half a cup of one of the above-mentioned herbal teas. Take half of this dose before breakfast and the other half after breakfast.

ANGINA PECTORIS

Agrimony Tea
Drink two cups of agrimony tea* every day, making sure that you sip it slowly.

Arnica Tincture
Massaging the area around the heart with arnica tincture* brings immediate relief. Take care to rub the tincture in very gently.

Hawthorn Tea
Drink two cups of hawthorn tea* in the course of the day, taking care to sip it slowly.

Hawthorn Tincture
Take between four and ten drops of hawthorn tincture* every day.

Heart Tonic
Use only additive-free biologically-produced wine for making this tonic. Pour 2 pt (1l) of wine into a saucepan and add twelve fresh parsley stems (leaves and all) and one to two tablespoons of pure wine vinegar. Bring this mixture to a boil and then turn down the heat and let it simmer gently for ten minutes. Strain off the parsley and stir in 12 oz (300g) of natural, unprocessed honey. Take two to three tablespoons of this tonic wine every day. You can make the tonic with white wine or red wine as you wish, it is purely a question of taste and the color has no effect on the potency of the tonic.

Swedish Bitters
Massage the area around your heart with undiluted Swedish bitters* several times a day.

Yarrow Tea
Drink two cups of yarrow tea* a day, taking care to sip it slowly.

APPENDIX (grumbling)

Raspberry Leaf Tea
Drink one or two cups of raspberry leaf tea* a day, taking care to sip it slowly. Continue to take the raspberry leaf tea until the irritation has subsided.

ARTERIOSCLEROSIS

Hawthorn Tea
Drink two cups of hawthorn tea* during the day, making sure that you sip it slowly.

Hawthorn Tincture
Take between four and ten drops of hawthorn tincture* every day.

Mistletoe Tea
Drink two to three cups of mistletoe tea* every day as a preventive measure, sipping it slowly. It's a good idea to keep your day's supply in a pre-warmed thermos.

Ramsons (Broad-leaved Garlic) Tincture
Taken regularly, ramsons tincture* can help to prevent arteriosclerosis. Take between ten and twelve drops four times a day in a little water.

Speedwell and Horsetail Tea

This tea can also help to prevent arteriosclerosis. Mix equal quantities of speedwell and horsetail and use one heaping teaspoonful of this mixture for each cup of tea. Pour on hot water and let the herbs steep for thirty seconds before straining them off. Drink one or two cups of this tea a day, taking care to sip it slowly.

If you're taking the tea as a preventive measure, it's perfectly all right to drink it the whole year round, but in such cases one cup a day is sufficient.

Speedwell Tea

Drink one to two cups of speedwell tea* a day, taking care to sip it slowly. Tea made from fresh speedwell is a particularly good preventive measure against arteriosclerosis, and it's a good idea to give yourself a treatment with it once a year.

ARTHRITIS

Calendula Ointment

This calendula ointment should be rubbed into the skin before you apply the Swedish bitters compresses (see below).

Melt 8 oz (250g) of pure lard in a saucepan and add two generous handfuls of calendula leaves, flowers and stems. Proceed according to the standard calendula ointment* recipe.

Comfrey Root Tincture

Comfrey root tincture helps to reduce the pain caused by arthritis. Massage it gently into the affected joints every day.

Horsetail Sitz Baths

Take one horsetail sitz bath* every month. The water should be just deep enough to cover your kidneys. Stay in the bath for twenty minutes, and don't dry yourself off when you get out; put on a dressing gown and get straight into bed, staying there for an hour so that you work up a good sweat.

Horsetail Tea

Drink two cups of horsetail tea* a day — one half an hour before breakfast in the morning and the other in the evening, half an hour before supper.

Leaf Poultices

Press some cabbage leaves (either savoy cabbage or white cabbage) with an iron until they are really hot, then wrap them around the affected joints, binding them into place with a clean cloth.

A poultice of club moss leaves is even more effective than cabbage leaves. Wash the freshly-picked leaves and then crush them on a wooden chopping board using a rolling pin. Apply the pulp directly to the affected joint and cover it gently with a clean cloth. It's best to apply this poultice in the evening and to leave it on overnight.

Nettle Tea

It's also a good idea to drink four cups of nettle tea* during the day, between the two cups of horsetail tea (see above). Drink the tea slowly, one sip at a time.

Swedish Bitters

Take three tablespoons of Swedish bitters* a day, dissolving each tablespoonful in half a cup of the nettle tea. Divide each of these three doses into two portions and take one of them before eating and the other one afterward.

Apply a Swedish bitters compress to the affected area once a day, leaving it on for four hours. Rub some of the calendula ointment into the joint first so that the alcohol in the Swedish bitters doesn't draw the natural oils out of your skin, and then moisten a large wad of cotton wool with the bitters and wrap it around the joint, covering it with a layer of dry cotton wool to retain the heat and a layer of plastic film to protect your clothes, then gently bind it all into place with a clean cloth. To prevent any skin irritation, dust your skin with a little talcum powder when you remove the compress.

ARTHROSIS

See Arthritis.

ASTHMA

Coltsfoot Juice

This juice is made by processing freshly-picked, washed coltsfoot leaves in a juice extractor. Take a teaspoonful of fresh coltsfoot juice two or three times a day in a cup of meat broth or warm milk.

Swedish Bitters Compresses

In my experience asthma is often caused by liver disorders. The liver becomes swollen and exerts pressure on the other organs, and this results in typical asthmatic symptoms. In such cases I recommend the application of Swedish Bitters* compresses.

Apply some calendula ointment* before you put on the compress so that the alcohol in the Bitters doesn't draw the natural oils out of your skin. Then moisten a wad of cotton wool with the Bitters and lay it over your liver, covering it with a dry wad of cotton wool to keep the warmth in and a layer of plastic film to protect your clothes. Bind everything into place with a warm cloth. Depending on how you feel, you can leave the compress on for up to four hours. If it feels comfortable, you can also apply it in the evening before going to sleep and leave it on overnight.

BLADDER (diseases of)

Agrimony Tea
Drink three cups of agrimony tea* in the course of the day, taking care to sip it slowly.

Chamomile Compresses
Pour some hot water into a bowl containing a handful of chamomile flowers. Then drain the flowers, wrap them in a clean linen cloth and lay them directly over your bladder, binding them gently into place with a warm cloth.

Club Moss Compresses
A dried club moss compress brings fast and sure relief from bladder spasms. Fill a pillowcase or small cushion cover with between 4 and 12 oz (100-300g) of dried club moss (depending on the size of the area that is feeling cramped), heat it up gently in the oven and apply it to your bladder in the evening, leaving it on overnight.

Golden Rod Tea
Golden rod has a diuretic effect, which makes it very useful for treating all kinds of bladder diseases. Drink up to four cups of golden rod tea* a day, making sure that you sip it slowly.

Herbal Mixture
Take equal measures of thyme and plantain and mix them well. Drink one to two cups of tea made from this mixture every day. To make the tea, use one heaping teaspoonful of the mixture for each cup, pour on hot water and let the herbs steep for thirty seconds before straining them off. Drink it slowly, one sip at a time.

Horsetail Vapor Treatment
Put a bowl containing four teaspoonfuls of horsetail on the floor and pour in 2 pt of hot water. Then put on a dressing gown and crouch down over the bowl, allowing the horsetail vapors to act on your bladder for ten minutes. You can also use the hot horsetail to make a compress, wrapping it up in a clean linen cloth and applying it directly over your bladder.

Willow-Herb Tea
Drink two cups of willow-herb tea* a day — one in the morning before breakfast and one in the evening, half an hour before supper. Take care to sip the tea slowly.

BLADDER (stones in)

Cowslip Root Tea
Drink one to two cups of cowslip root tea* a day, taking care to sip it slowly.

Horsetail Sitz Baths
A good way of obtaining very speedy relief from bladder stones is to drink horsetail tea while taking a horsetail sitz bath*. This combination stimulates the functioning of the bladder, and for the treatment to be effective you should refrain from urinating for as long as you can. This builds up the pressure in the bladder, which helps to wash the stones out of your urinary tract when you eventually empty your bladder.

Stay in the bath for twenty minutes, and don't dry yourself off when you get out; put on a robe and get straight into bed. Stay there for an hour so that you work up a good sweat. Drink between one and two cups of horsetail tea* while you are taking your sitz bath. Drink the tea slowly, one sip at a time.

Plantain Seeds
Plantain seeds are a traditional remedy for all kinds of stones. Take ¼ oz (8g) of these seeds a day, washing them down with a cup of plantain tea*. Take the seeds a little at a time, washing each portion down with a mouthful of the tea.

BLADDER (weakness of)

Knotgrass Root Tea
Use one heaping teaspoonful of knotgrass root for each cup of tea and soak it in the cold water for twelve hours. Then heat the infusion up gently and strain it. Drink four cups of this tea over a day,

taking care to sip it slowly. It's a good idea to keep your day's supply in a pre-warmed thermos.

Lady's Mantle Tea
Drink four cups of lady's mantle tea* in the course of the day, sipping it slowly.

Salt-Water Baths
Salt-water baths are a traditional and very effective remedy for weakness of the bladder. Dissolve a handful of ordinary household salt in your bathwater, which should be pleasantly warm and just deep enough to cover your kidneys. Stay in the bath for twenty minutes, and don't dry yourself off when you get out; put on a robe and get straight into bed. Stay there for an hour so that you work up a good sweat.

Shepherd's Purse Tincture
Massaging the bladder area with shepherd's purse tincture* helps to improve muscle tone. Gently massage the area around your bladder with the tincture several times a day.

Sitz Baths
Shepherd's purse, yarrow and horsetail sitz baths are all excellent remedies for atony of the bladder.

Take 4 oz (100g) of one of these herbs for each bath and soak them in 1 gal (5l) of cold water for twelve hours. Then heat the infusion up gently and strain the liquid into your bathwater. The water should be just deep enough to cover your kidneys. Stay in the bath for twenty minutes, and don't dry yourself off when you get out; put on a dressing gown and get straight into bed, staying there for an hour so that you work up a good sweat. If you wish you can also make a mixture of equal parts of shepherd's purse, yarrow and horsetail and use this for preparing your baths.

BLEEDING

Horsetail Tea
Horsetail staunches bleeding very effectively. It can be used to treat uterine, pulmonary, and gastric hemorrhages, and also bleeding hemorrhoids. Use two to three heaping teaspoons of horsetail for each cup of tea, pour on hot water and let the horsetail steep for thirty seconds before straining it off. Drink two or three cups of tea a day (depending on the severity of the hemorrhage), taking care to sip it slowly.

Mistletoe Tea
The ability to mistletoe to normalize both high and low blood-pressure makes it very useful for the treatment of excessive menstrual bleeding. Drink one to three cups of mistletoe tea* every day (depending on the severity of the bleeding), sipping it slowly. It's a good idea to keep your day's supply in a pre-warmed thermos.

Shepherd's Purse Tea
Shepherd's purse tea* also helps to staunch bleeding. Drink two to three cups during the day, taking care to sip it slowly.

BLOOD CHOLESTEROL LEVEL (high)

Speedwell Tea
A high blood cholesterol level can be brought down with the help of speedwell tea*. Drink two cups a day, taking care to sip it slowly.

BONES (fractures)

Lady's Mantle Tea
Drink two cups of lady's mantle tea* in the course of the day, taking care to sip it slowly.

Mallow Foot and Hand Baths
If you have a fractured bone in one of your hands or feet the painful swelling can be reduced by bathing them in a mallow wash*. Soak the hand or foot in the liquid for twenty minutes.

BREAST (lumps)

(N.B. At the first sign of such lumps professional advice should be sought.)

Calendula Ointment
Breast lumps can be treated externally with calendula ointment. Gently rub the ointment into the breast every day. If an operation has already been carried out you can apply the ointment to the scars. The strained-off residue from making the ointment can be heated up again and used to make a warm compress, which helps to smooth the skin. You can use this residue four to five times before throwing it away.

Melt 8 oz (250g) of pure lard in a saucepan and

add two generous handfuls of calendula leaves, flowers and stems. Proceed according to the standard recipe for calendula ointment*

BRONCHIAL ASTHMA

Coltsfoot Leaf Juice
Coltsfoot juice can only be made in the spring, when the plants are ripe. Wash some freshly-picked coltsfoot leaves carefully and process them in a juice extractor. Take a teaspoonful of fresh coltsfoot leaf juice two to three times a day, dissolving it in a cup of meat broth or warm milk.

Coltsfoot Tea
Drink two to three cups of coltsfoot tea* a day, taking care to sip it slowly.

Plantain and Thyme Tea
Drink the plantain and thyme tea* as hot as you can bear it, one sip at a time. Take between four and five cups of this tea a day, making each cup fresh just before you drink it.

BURSITIS

Coltsfoot Compresses
Wash some freshly-picked coltsfoot leaves and crush them to a pulp on a wooden chopping board using a rolling pin. Apply the pulp to a clean linen cloth and wrap it around the affected area.

Horsetail Compresses
Put two generous handfuls of horsetail in a sieve and heat it up over boiling water. When the horsetail is really hot, wrap it up in a clean linen cloth and wrap it around the affected area, binding it gently into place with another cloth to keep the heat in. Leave the compress on for two hours.

Horsetail Sitz Baths
The horsetail sitz bath* water should be just deep enough to cover your kidneys. Stay in the bath for twenty minutes, and don't dry yourself off when you get out; put on a robe and get straight into bed. Stay there for an hour so that you work up a good sweat.

Horsetail Tea
Horsetail can also be taken internally as a tea. Drink two cups of horsetail tea* a day — one in the morning and the other in the evening — taking care to sip it slowly.

Mallow Tea
Drink up to four cups of mallow tea* in the course of the day, taking care to sip it slowly. It's a good idea to keep your day's supply in a pre-warmed thermos.

Swedish Bitters Compresses
Swedish bitters compresses are another good external remedy for bursitis. Moisten a wad of cotton wool with Swedish bitters* and apply it to the affected area, covering it with a layer of dry cotton wool and a layer of plastic film to keep the warmth in. Bind everything gently into place with a warm cloth.

CATARACTS

As I see it both grey cataracts and glaucomas are more than simple eye diseases — in many cases they are also associated with a dysfunction of the kidneys.

Celandine Juice
Never apply the thick juice from the flower stems of the celandine to your eyes, use only the juice from the leafstems! Take a freshly-picked celandine leaf, wash it thoroughly and crush the stem between your fingers without drying it off first. Apply the juice directly to your eyelids with your fingers, keeping your eyes closed as you do so. Repeat this procedure several times a day.

Before you go to sleep at night, it's a good idea to place freshly-washed celandine leaves over your eyes, binding, them gently into place with a warm cloth.

Eyebright Tea
Use no more than half a teaspoonful of eyebright for each cupful of tea. Pour on hot water and let the eyebright steep for ten seconds before straining it off. Rinse your eyes out thoroughly with this tea (let it cool first!), using an ordinary eyebath from the chemist's.

If you find that these eyebaths disagree with you, you can apply eyebright compresses instead. Soak a clean cloth in the tea and lay it over your eyes. It is important to make this tea fresh every time you use it.

Herbal Mixture
Mix equal quantities of stinging nettles, speedwell, calendula and horsetail. Drink two to three cups

of tea brewed from this mixture a day. Use one heaping teaspoonful of the mixture for each cup of tea. Pour on hot water and let the herbs steep for thirty seconds before straining them off. Drink the tea slowly, one sip at a time.

Use fresh herbs if at all possible, as they are more potent than the dried ones.

Horsetail Sitz Baths

Horsetail sitz baths* are particularly helpful if you suffer from glaucoma, as this disease is often caused by distended, poorly-functioning kidneys. The water should be just deep enough to cover your kidneys. Stay in the bath for twenty minutes, and don't dry yourself off when you get out; put on a robe and get straight into bed. Stay there for an hour so that you work up a good sweat.

Swedish Bitters

Take three teaspoons of Swedish bitters* a day, dissolving each teaspoonful in half a cup of the mixed herb tea described above. Divide each of these three doses into two portions, taking one of them before eating and the other one afterwards.

You can also use Swedish bitters externally, applying it directly to your eyelids with your fingers. Keep your eye closed when you do this, and stroke outward from the root of your nose toward the corners of your eyes.

Vapor Baths

Mix ½ oz (10g) of eyebright, ¾ oz (20g) of valerian, ½ oz (10g) of verbena, 1½ oz (30g) of elderflowers and ¾ oz (20g) of chamomile. Pour 1 pt (½l) of hot white wine into a bowl containing five level teaspoonfuls of this herbal mixture. Hold your head over the bowl and allow the vapors to act on your closed eyes. Transfer the wine and herb mixture to a bottle when you have finished — if you heat it up again you can make a total of three vapor baths with the same batch.

COLIC

Calamus Root Tea

The root of the calamus also has purifying properties, helping to clean out the stomach and the intestines.

Drink one mouthful of calamus root tea* before and after each meal, i.e., a total of six mouthfuls a day. This is equivalent to one cup, and it is important not to drink more than this quantity in any one day. It's a good idea to keep your day's supply in a pre-warmed thermos.

Horsetail Compresses

Put two heaping handfuls of horsetail in a sieve and heat it up over boiling water. When the horsetail is really hot, wrap it up in a clean linen cloth and apply it to your abdomen, binding it with another cloth to keep the heat in. Leave the compress on for several hours, or apply it in the evening before going to bed and leave it on overnight.

Ramsons (Broad-leaved Garlic)

The blood-purifying properties of ramsons make it an excellent remedy for gastric and intestinal colic, bringing speedy relief.

Fresh ramsons leaves can be collected in the spring and should be eaten raw. Wash them, chop them up finely, and sprinkle them on your food as you would fresh parsley. Spinach tastes lovely if you cook it with a few ramsons leaves, and they also make an excellent addition to salads.

Swedish Bitters

Swedish bitters* are a good remedy for fits of colic. Take one tablespoonful three times a day in a little water or herb tea.

Swedish Bitters Compresses

I can personally vouch for the fact that Swedish bitters* compresses bring speedy relief from renal colic. Apply some calendula ointment* before putting on the compress to prevent the alcohol in the bitters from drawing the natural oils out of your skin. Then moisten a wad of cotton wool with Swedish bitters and place it over your kidneys, covering it with a layer of dry cotton wool and a layer of plastic film to keep in the warmth. Bind everything in place with a warm cloth and leave the compress on for four hours.

COLITIS

Calendula Tea

Drink two cups of calendula tea* a day, taking care to sip it slowly.

Mallow Tea

Soak two heaping teaspoons of mallow in two cups of cold water for twelve hours. Then heat up the infusion gently and strain off the mallow. Make the two cups of tea last the whole day, taking little sips at regular intervals.

CORNEA (opacities or flecks in)

Celandine Juice
Never use the thick juice from the flower stems of the celandine for treating your eyes! Only use the juice from the leafstems. Wash a freshly-picked leafstem carefully, crush it between your moistened fingers and apply the juice directly to your eyelids with your fingers. Start at the root of your nose and stroke outward toward the corners of your eyes, keeping your eyes closed. In the evening, before you go to bed, it's a good idea to place some fresh celandine leaves over your eyes (wash the leaves first), binding them into place with a clean cloth.

CYSTS

Horsetail Compresses
Put two generous handfuls of horsetail in a sieve and heat it up over boiling water. When the horsetail is really hot, wrap it up in a clean linen cloth and apply it to the cyst, binding it gently into place with another cloth to keep the heat in.

Apply three of these hot horsetail compresses every day. You can use the same batch of horsetail for all three compresses, heating it up again every time you use it.

The first compress should be applied in the morning before rising, the second in the late afternoon and the third at night, directly before going to sleep. Stay in bed for two hours after putting the first two compresses on so that they have a chance to work properly, and leave the third compress on overnight. It is very important to bind a thick, warm cloth around the compresses and to wrap yourself up as warmly as possible so that the healing horsetail vapors are not wasted.

Swedish Bitters Compresses
You should apply a Swedish bitters compress around midday, between the first horsetail compress and the second, and leave it on for four hours. Apply a little calendula ointment (see below) before putting on the compress to prevent the alcohol in the bitters from drawing the natural oils out of your skin. Then moisten a wad of cotton wool with Swedish bitters* and lay it over the cyst, covering it with a layer of dry cotton wool to keep the warmth in and a layer of plastic film to protect your clothes. Finally, bind everything gently into place with a clean cloth. When the four hours are up, remove the compress and dust the skin with a little talcum powder to prevent any possible irritation.

There is no need to stay in bed while you have the Swedish bitters compress on, but do remain indoors.

Horsetail Tea
As a supplement to the compresses you should also take two cups of horsetail tea* every day — one before breakfast and the other before your evening meal. Drink the tea slowly, one sip at a time.

Herbal Mixture
Mix 4 oz (100g) of stinging nettles, 12 oz (300g) of calendula and 4 oz (100g) of yarrow. In addition to the treatment with the compresses and the horsetail tea, drink 2½ to 3½ pt (1½-2l) of tea brewed from this mixture every day.

Use one heaping teaspoonful of the mixture for each cup of tea. Pour on hot water and let the herbs steep for thirty seconds before straining them off. Drink the tea slowly, one sip at a time.

If it's available you should also take between three and five drops of sorrel juice six times a day, dissolving each of the six doses in a cup of the mixed herb tea. To make the juice simply wash some fresh common sorrel and run it through a juice extractor.

Calendula Ointment
The calendula ointment that should be applied to the skin before putting on the Swedish bitters compresses is made as follows.

First melt 8 oz (250g) of pure lard in a saucepan and then add two generous handfuls of calendula leaves, flowers and stems. Proceed according to the standard recipe for calendula ointment*.

EMPHYSEMA

Emphysema is the term used to describe a pathological condition in which air collects in a tissue or organ. This is often caused by disorders of the livers.

Club Moss Tea
Drink one cup of club moss tea* a day, taking half of it before breakfast and half of it afterward. Sip it slowly.

Horsetail Compresses

Apply a hot horsetail compress to your liver in the evening and leave it on overnight.

Put two generous handfuls of horsetail in a sieve and heat it up over boiling water, taking care that the sieve does not actually come into contact with the water. Once the horsetail is really hot, wrap it up in a clean linen cloth and place it over your liver, binding it gently into place with a warm cloth.

Swedish Bitters Compresses

Cases of emphysema caused by disorders of the liver can also be treated with Swedish bitters* compresses.

Apply some calendula ointment* before putting on the compress so that the alcohol in the bitters doesn't draw the natural oils out of the skin. Then moisten a large wad of cotton wool with Swedish bitters and lay it over your liver, covering it with a layer of dry cotton wool to keep the warmth in and a layer of plastic film to protect your clothes. Bind everything into place with a warm cloth and leave the compress on for four hours.

FEET (varicose ulcers on)

Calendula Ointment

After bathing your feet apply some calendula ointment* around the edges of the ulcers.

Calendula and Horsetail Wash

Mix equal quantities of calendula and horsetail. Pour 1 pt (½l) of hot water into a bowl containing two heaping tablespoonfuls of this mixture and let it steep for thirty seconds before straining it. Bathe the affected area gently with the lukewarm liquid.

Horsetail Footbaths

Bathing your feet in this horsetail infusion helps to reduce the swelling caused by varicose ulcers. Pour 1 pt (½l) of hot water into a bowl containing two heaping tablespoons of horsetail and let it steep for twenty minutes before straining it. Bathe your feet in the undiluted infusion for twenty minutes.

Mallow Footbaths

Use the standard recipe for a mallow wash* and bathe your feet in the liquid for twenty minutes. Mallow footbaths are particularly good for swollen feet.

Plantain Leaf Dressings

After taking a footbath, apply fresh plantain leaf dressings to the ulcers. Wash some freshly-picked plantain leaves, crush them to a pulp on a wooden chopping board using a rolling pin (don't dry the leaves off first) and apply the pulp directly to the affected areas.

FISTULAS

A fistula is an abnormal pipe-shaped opening between one hollow organ and another or between a hollow organ and the surface of the skin.

Calendula Ointment

Calendula ointment* is a good external remedy for fistulas. You can also make warm compresses with the strained calendula residue. This can be heated up again and used a total of three times before it is thrown away.

Horsetail Compresses

Apply a hot horsetail compress in the evening and leave it on overnight. Put two heaping handfuls of horsetail in a sieve and heat it up over boiling water, taking care that the sieve does not actually come into contact with the water. Once the horsetail is really hot, wrap it up in a clean linen cloth and apply it to the affected area, binding it into place with a warm cloth.

Horsetail Sitz Baths

The healing of fistulas can be speeded up by taking regular horsetail sitz baths*. The water should be just deep enough to cover your kidneys. Stay in the bath for twenty minutes, and don't dry yourself off when you get out; put on a robe and get straight into bed, staying there for an hour so that you work up a good sweat.

Horsetail and St John's Wort Tea

Fistulas in the palate or the throat can be treated by gargling with a herb tea made with a mixture of equal quantities of horsetail and St John's wort. Use one heaping teaspoonful of this mixture for each cup of tea. Pour on hot water and let the herbs steep for thirty seconds before straining them off. Gargle with the tea several times a day.

Mixed Herb Wash

Soak equal quantities of ground ivy, linaria and

horsetail in cold water for twelve hours. Then heat up the infusion gently and strain it. Bathe the affected area with the warm liquid, repeating the process every day, and dab a little Swedish bitters* on to the area around the fistula with a wad of cotton wool afterwards.

Nettle Tea
Drink three cups of nettle tea* a day, taking care to sip it slowly.

Swedish Bitters
Take one teaspoonful of Swedish bitters* three times a day in a little of the nettle tea*. Divide each of these three doses into two portions, taking one portion before eating and the other one afterwards.

FROSTBITE

Calamus Root Wash
Soak 4 oz (100g) of calamus root in 1 gal (5l) of water for twelve hours. Then heat up the infusion gently and strain it. Bathe the affected areas in the warm wash for twenty minutes.

Mistletoe Berry Ointment
This ointment is a good treatment for frostbite. You make it by blending fresh mistletoe berries with cold lard. (N.B. Do not take internally. Mistletoe berries are poisonous.)

Mistletoe Wash
Soak a handful of fresh mistletoe leaves in 1 gal (5l) of cold water for twelve hours. Then heat up the infusion gently and strain it. Bathe the affected areas in the warm liquid for twenty minutes.

You can also make a dressing from freshly-picked mistletoe leaves. Wash the leaves, crush them to a pulp on a wooden chopping board using a rolling pin and apply the pulp directly to the affected areas.

Swedish Bitters Compresses
Swedish bitters* compresses are another effective remedy for frostbite. Apply some calendula ointment* before you put on the compress so that the alcohol in the bitters doesn't draw the natural oils out of your skin. Then moisten a wad of cotton wool with Swedish bitters and apply it to the affected area, covering it with a layer of dry cotton wool to keep in the warmth and a layer of plastic film to protect your clothes. Bind everything into place with a warm cloth.

GALL-BLADDER
(biliary colic)

Horsetail Compresses
Hot horsetail compresses can bring speedy relief from attacks of biliary colic, which can often be extremely painful.

Put two heaping handfuls of horsetail in a sieve and heat it up over boiling water. When the horsetail is really hot, wrap it in a clean linen cloth and apply it over your gall-bladder, binding it into place with a warm cloth.

Swedish Bitters Compresses
If the attack of biliary colic is severe, it is advisable to apply a Swedish bitters* compress. Apply some calendula ointment* before you put the compress on so that the alcohol in the bitters doesn't draw the natural oils out of your skin. Then moisten a wad of cotton wool with bitters and apply it over your gall-bladder, covering it with a layer of dry cotton wool to keep the warmth in and a layer of plastic film to protect your clothes. Bind everything into place with a warm cloth and leave the compress on for four hours.

GALL-BLADDER
(diseases of)

Calamus Root Tea
Drink one mouthful of calamus root tea* before and after each meal, i.e., a total of six mouthfuls a day (this is equivalent to one cup). It's a good idea to keep your day's supply in a pre-warmed thermos.

Dandelion Stems
Eat between five and six raw, freshly-picked dandelion stems every day, washing them carefully beforehand and chewing them very thoroughly. Don't cut off the flowers until after you have washed the plants. The dandelions must be picked while they are in flower.

Nettle Tea
If you have any kind of bladder disease or complaint it's a good idea to give yourself a proper treatment with nettle tea, drinking up to four cups a day for several weeks. Drink the tea slowly, one sip at a time.

Wild Chicory Root Tea
Drink two cups of wild chicory root tea* in the

course of the day. It's a good idea to keep your day's supply in a pre-warmed thermos.

GALLSTONES

Cider Tonic
Mix equal quantities (by weight) of pimpernel, ivy, hops, peppermint, agrimony and wormwood. Soak three tablespoonfuls of this mixture in 2 pt (1l) of still cider for twelve hours. Then heat the cider up gently until it comes to the boil, remove the pot from the heat and let the herbs steep for thirty seconds before straining them off. Transfer the tonic to a thermos before it cools, and take one tablespoonful eight times a day at hourly intervals.

Dandelion Stems
In some cases a treatment with dandelion stems can be enough to dissolve gallstones easily and painlessly. Eat between five and six raw, freshly-picked dandelion stems every day, washing them carefully beforehand and chewing them very thoroughly. Don't cut off the flowers until after you have washed the plants. This treatment is only possible in the spring, as the dandelions must be picked while they are in flower.

Herbal Mixture
Mix equal quantities (by weight) of birch leaves, restharrow, shepherd's purse and agrimony. Drink two cups of tea brewed from this mixture every day, using one heaping teaspoonful for each cup. Pour on hot water, let the herbs steep for thirty seconds before straining them off and drink the tea slowly, one sip at a time.

Plantain Tea
Drink up to three cups of plantain tea* a day, taking care to sip it slowly.

It's also a good idea to take a total of ¼ oz (8g) of plantain seeds in the course of the day, washing them down with the plantain tea, as this can help to prevent the formation of new stones.

Radish Juice
A six-week course of treatment with fresh radish juice is an effective traditional remedy for gallstones. To make the juice, wash and peel the radishes (use the large, long, white variety, not the small red garden radish) and run them through a juice extractor. Start with 3½ fl oz (100ml) of juice a day, increasing the quantity slowly to 14 fl oz (400ml) by the end of the first three weeks. Reduce

the quantity again after this, cutting it down progressively so that you reach 3½ fl oz (100ml) a day again at the end of the second three weeks. Always drink the juice on an empty stomach.

This course of treatment is not suitable for people who have gastric or intestinal disorders.

GLANDS (diseases of)

Calamus Root Tea
Drink one mouthful of calamus flat root tea* before and after each meal. It's important not to drink more than one cupful in any one day.

Calamus Leaf Dressings
Serious cases of adenopathy can be treated with the help of dressings made from crushed plantain or great plantain leaves. Wash some freshy-picked leaves, crush them to a pulp on a wooden chopping board using a rolling pin and apply the pulp directly to the affected glands.

Mistletoe Tea
Drink up to three cups of mistletoe tea* every day, taking care to sip it slowly. It's a good idea to keep your day's supply in a pre-warmed thermos.

Sage Tea
Drink two cups of sage tea* a day, taking care to sip it slowly.

GLANDS (swollen)

Calendula Wash
Pour 1 pt (½l) of hot water into a bowl containing one heaping tablespoonful of calendula and let it steep for half an hour before straining it. Bathe the swollen glands with the wash.

Dandelion Stems
Eat between ten and twelve raw, freshly-picked dandelion stems every day for three to four weeks, washing them carefully beforehand and chewing them very thoroughly. Don't cut off the flowers until after you have washed the plants. This treatment is only possible in the spring, as the dandelions must be picked while they are still in flower.

St John's Wort Oil
Use St John's wort oil* as an embrocation, applying it directly to the swollen glands.

GOITER

Figwort Tea
Use one heaping teaspoonful of finely-chopped fresh figwort leaves for each cup of tea. Pour on hot water and let the herbs steep for thirty seconds before straining them off. Gargle with this tea several times a day, taking great care not to swallow it.

Bedstraw Tea
Bedstraw tea* also makes an effective gargle for treating goiter. Gargle with it several times a day, swallowing a mouthful of the tea every now and then.

Plantain Poultices
Wash some fresh plantain leaves, crush them between your fingers, mix them with a little salt and apply the mixture directly to your neck, binding it gently into place with a clean cloth.

HEART (cardiac asthma)

Calendula Ointment
This calendula ointment should be rubbed into the skin before you apply the Swedish bitters compresses (see below).

Melt 8 oz (250g) of pure lard in a saucepan and add four generous handfuls of calendula leaves, flowers and stems. Proceed according to the standard calendula ointment* recipe.

Club Moss Tea
Drink one cup of club moss tea* in the morning and another in the evening, taking care to sip it slowly.

Horsetail Compresses
Apply a hot horsetail poultice in the evening and leave it on overnight.

Put a generous handful of horsetail in a sieve and heat it up over boiling water. When the horsetail is really hot, wrap it up in a clean linen cloth, apply it over your liver and bind it gently into place with another warm cloth.

Swedish Bitters
Take one teaspoonful of Swedish bitters* with each of the cups of club moss tea (see above).

Swedish Bitters Compresses
During the daytime it's advisable to supplement the effects of the hot horsetail poultices (see above) with a Swedish bitters compress, which should be applied over the liver in the same way as the horsetail poultices.

Apply some calendula ointment first to prevent the alcohol in the bitters from drawing the natural oils out of your skin. Then moisten a wad of cotton wool with Swedish bitters and lay it over your liver, covering it with a layer of dry cotton wool and a layer of plastic film to keep the warmth in. Bind everything into place with a warm cloth and leave the compress on for four hours.

Hawthorn Tincture
Take between four and ten drops of hawthorn tincture* every day.

Ramsons Juice
Wash some fresh ramsons leaves and run them through a juice extractor. Apply the fresh juice directly to the area around the heart.

HEART (coronary vasoconstriction)

Arnica Tincture
Massaging the area around the heart gently with arnica tincture* brings speedy relief from constriction of the coronary vessels and nervous heart disorders.

Nettle Tea
Pour 2 pt (1l) of hot water into a bowl containing four heaping teaspoonfuls of stinging nettles and let them steep for thirty seconds before sieving them off. Bathe the area around the heart with the lukewarm tea, massaging it gently at the same time.

HEART (palpitations)

Hawthorn Tea
Drink two cups of hawthorn tea* in the course of the day, taking care to sip it slowly.

Hawthorn Tincture
Take between four and ten drops of hawthorn tincture* every day.

Mistletoe Tea
Drink three cups of mistletoe tea* in the course of the day, taking care to sip it slowly. It's a good

idea to keep your day's supply in a pre-warmed thermos.

HERNIAS

Lady's Mantle Tea
If at all possible, you should use fresh lady's mantle for making this tea. Drink four cups of lady's mantle tea* in the course of the day, taking care to sip it slowly.

Shepherd's Purse Tincture
Gently massage a little shepherd's purse tincture* into the hernia several times a day.

HYSTERIA

Bedstraw Tea
Drink two to three cups of bedstraw tea* in the course of the day, taking care to sip it slowly.

Mistletoe Tea
Drink three cups of mistletoe tea* in the course of the day, taking care to sip it slowly. It's a good idea to keep your day's supply in a pre-warmed thermos.

St John's Wort Sitz Baths
Soak 4 oz (100g) of St John's wort in 1 gal (5l) of cold water for twelve hours. When the time is up heat up the infusion gently and strain it into your bathwater. The water should be just deep enough to cover your kidneys. Stay in the bath for twenty minues, and don't dry yourself off when you get out; put on a robe and get straight into bed. Stay there for an hour so that you work up a good sweat.

St John's Wort Tea
Drink two cups of St John's wort tea* in the course of the day, taking care to sip it slowly.

INFERTILITY

Mistletoe Juice
Women who are unable to have children should take twenty-five drops of mistletoe juice twice a day. Take the first dose in the morning before breakfast and the second at night, just before going to sleep. Mistletoe juice is available at drug stores and health food shops, but it is easy to make at home. All you need to do is to wash some freshly-picked mistletoe leaves thoroughly and then run it through a juice extractor. (**N.B. Mistletoe berries are poisonous.**)

INTERVERTEBRAL DISCS (damaged)

Comfrey Baths
If you have slipped or damaged discs it's helpful to take frequent comfrey baths.

Soak either 1 lb (500g) of fresh or 6½ oz (200g) of dried comfrey leaves in 1 gal (5l) of cold water for twelve hours. Then heat up the infusion gently and strain the liquid into your bathwater. It's important that your heart should stay above the water level. Stay in the bath for twenty minutes, and don't dry yourself off when you get out; put on a robe and get straight into bed. Stay there for an hour so that you work up a good sweat.

Horsetail Sitz Baths
The water in your horsetail sitz bath* should be just deep enough to cover your kidneys. Stay in the bath for twenty minutes, and don't dry yourself off when you get out; put on a robe and get straight into bed. Stay there for an hour so that you work up a good sweat.

INTERVERTEBRAL DISCS (disorders of)

Horsetail Sitz Baths
Horsetail sitz baths* bring amazingly rapid relief from disc disorders. The water should be just deep enough to cover your kidneys. Stay in the bath for twenty minutes, and don't dry yourself off when you get out; put on a robe and get straight into bed. Stay there for an hour so that you work up a good sweat.

Peony Root Baths
Take two heaping handfuls of peony roots, wash them, grate them and soak the grated roots in 1 gal (5l) of cold water for twelve hours. Then heat the infusion up gently and strain it into your bathwater. It is important that your heart should stay above the water level. Sit in the bath for twenty minutes, and don't dry yourself off when you get out; put on a robe and get straight into bed. Stay

there for an hour so that you work up a good sweat.

Peony Root Tincture

Peony root baths are even more effective if you add three tablespoons of peony root tincture to the water. Wash and grate enough peony roots to fill the bottle you wish to use and put them into the bottle. Then add enough 38-40% grain alcohol to cover the grated roots completely, seal the bottle and leave it to stand in a warm place for at least two weeks before using the tincture.

INTESTINAL ULCERS

Calendula Tea

Drink two cups of calendula tea* in the course of the day, taking care to sip it slowly.

Knotgrass Tea

Drink two cups of knotgrass tea* in the course of the day, making sure that you sip it slowly.

Mallow Leaves

Make yourself some barley soup and, just before you eat it, add some freshly-picked, finely-chopped mallow leaves. Don't boil the leaves with the soup as this will destroy some of the valuable mucin-rich substances that they contain.

Nettle Tea

Drink three or four cups of nettle tea* during the day, taking care to sip it slowly.

INTESTINE (prolapse of)

Lady's Mantle Tea

Drink four cups of lady's mantle tea* a day, taking care to sip it slowly.

Shepherd's Purse Tincture

Rub a little shepherd's purse tincture* into the skin around the anus several times a day.

Shepherd's purse tincture can also be taken internally. Take ten drops a day in a little lady's mantle tea*.

JAUNDICE

Celandine Wine

Wash 1 oz (30g) of celandine (including the roots) and soak it in 1 pt (½l) of dry white wine for two hours. Then strain off the celandine. Take one tablespoonful of celandine wine every hour during the daytime.

Dandelion Stems

The blood-purifying properties of the dandelion make it useful in the treatment of jaundice. Eat up to ten raw, freshly-picked dandelion stems every day, washing them carefully beforehand and chewing them very thoroughly. Don't cut off the flowers until after you have washed the plants. This treatment is only possible in the spring, as the dandelions must be picked while they are in flower.

Herbal Mixture

Mix 2 oz (50g) of speedwell, 2 oz (50g) of dandelion root, 1 oz (25g) of woodruff and 1 oz (25g) of wild chicory flowers. Drink two cups of tea brewed from this mixture every day. Use one heaping teaspoonful of the mixture for each cup of tea. Pour on hot water and let the herbs steep for thirty seconds before straining them off. Drink the tea slowly, one sip at a time.

Sorrel Tea

Drink two cups of sorrel tea* in the course of the day, taking care to sip it slowly.

Swedish Bitters

Take three tablespoons of Swedish bitters* a day, dissolving each tablespoonful in half a cup of one of the herb teas described here. Divide each of these three doses into two portions, taking one before eating and one afterwards.

Swedish Bitters Compresses

Swedish bitters compresses* on the liver are also helpful. Apply some calendula ointment* before you put on the compress to prevent the alcohol in the bitters from drawing the natural oils out of your skin. Then moisten a wad of cotton wool with Swedish bitters and apply it over your liver, covering it with a layer of dry cotton wool to keep the warmth in and a layer of plastic film to protect your clothes. Bind everything into place with a warm cloth and leave it on for four hours.

Walnut Leaf Tea

Drink two to three cups of walnut leaf tea* in the course of the day, taking care to sip it slowly.

Wild Chicory Tea

Drink two cups of wild chicory tea* during the day, taking care to sip it slowly. It's a good idea to keep your day's supply in a pre-warmed thermos.

JOINTS (attrition of)

Cabbage and Club Moss Poultices

Iron some cabbage leaves (either white cabbage or savoy cabbage) until they are really hot and apply them directly to the affected joints, binding them gently into place with a warm cloth.

Club moss poultices are even more effective. Take some freshly-picked club moss leaves, crush them to a pulp on a wooden chopping board using a rolling pin and apply the pulp directly to the affected joints, binding them with a warm cloth. It's best to apply the poultices in the evening and to leave them on overnight.

Comfrey Root Tincture

A regular gentle massage with comfrey root tincture* can help to reduce the pain caused by worn joints. Massage the affected joints with this tincture every day.

Horsetail Sitz Baths

Take one horsetail sitz bath* every month. The water should be just deep enough to cover your kidneys. Stay in the bath for twenty minutes, and don't dry yourself off when you get out; put on a robe and get straight into bed. Stay there for an hour so that you work up a good sweat.

Horsetail Tea

Drink two cups of horsetail tea* every day, one half an hour before breakfast in the morning and the other half an hour before supper in the evening.

Meadowsweet Tea

Drink two to three cups of meadowsweet tea* in the course of the day, taking care to sip it slowly.

Nettle Tea

In addition to horsetail tea it's also a good idea to take four cups of nettle tea* a day. Drink it one sip at a time during the daytime, between the two cups of horsetail tea.

Swedish Bitters

Take three tablespoons of Swedish bitters* a day, dissolving each tablespoonful in half a cup of the nettle tea*. Divide each of these three doses into two portions, taking one before eating and one afterwards.

Swedish Bitters Compresses

Apply some calendula ointment* before you put the compress on in order to prevent the alcohol in the bitters from drawing the natural oils out of your skin. Then moisten a wad of cotton wool with Swedish bitters* and wrap it around the joint, covering it with a layer of dry cotton wool to keep the warmth in and a layer of plastic film to protect your clothes. Bind everything into place with a clean cloth. Apply one Swedish bitters compress every day, leaving it on for four hours.

JOINTS (deformities of)

Cabbage and Club Moss Poultices

Iron some cabbage leaves (either white cabbage or savoy cabbage) until they are really hot and apply them directly to the affected joints, binding them into place with a warm cloth.

Club moss poultices are even more effective. Take some freshly-picked club moss leaves, crush them to a pulp on a wooden chopping board using a rolling pin and apply the pulp directly to the affected joints, binding them with a warm cloth. It's best to apply the poultices in the evening and to leave them on overnight.

Comfrey Root Tincture

A regular gentle massage with comfrey root tincture* can help to reduce the pain in the joints. Massage the affected joints with this tincture every day.

Horsetail Sitz Baths

Take one horsetail sitz bath* every month. The water should be just deep enough to cover your kidneys. Stay in the bath for twenty minutes, and don't dry yourself off when you get out; put on a robe and get straight into bed. Stay there for an hour so that you work up a good sweat.

Horsetail Tea

Drink two cups of horsetail tea* every day; one half an hour before breakfast in the morning and the other half an hour before supper in the evening.

Nettle Tea

In addition to horsetail tea it's also a good idea to take four cups of nettle tea* a day. Drink it during the daytime, between the two cups of horsetail tea, taking one sip at a time.

Swedish Bitters

Take three tablespoons of Swedish bitters* a day,

dissolving each tablespoonful in half a cup of the nettle tea*. Divide each of these three doses into two portions, taking one before eating and one afterward.

Swedish Bitters Compresses

Apply some calendula ointment* to the joint before you put the compress on so that the alcohol in the bitters doesn't draw the natural oils out of your skin. Then moisten a suitably large wad of cotton wool with Swedish bitters* and wrap it around the joint, covering it with a layer of dry cotton wool to keep the warmth in and a layer of plastic film to protect your clothes. Bind everything into place with a clean cloth. Apply one Swedish bitters compress to the affected area every day, leaving it on for four hours.

Dust the skin with a little talcum powder when you take the compresses off to prevent any possible irritation.

JOINTS (diseases of)

Club Moss Tea

Drink one cup of club moss tea* in the morning before breakfast, taking care to sip it slowly.

KIDNEYS (complaints of)

Horsetail Sitz Baths

The best variety of horsetail for these sitz baths is the great horsetail, which has thick stems and is found growing on mountain pastures and in marshy meadows.

The horsetail sitz bath* water should be just deep enough to cover your kidneys. Stay in the bath for twenty minutes, and don't dry yourself off when you get out; put on a robe and get straight into bed. Stay there for an hour so that you work up a good sweat.

Swedish Bitters

Take between three teaspoonfuls and three tablespoonfuls of Swedish bitters* a day (depending on the severity of the complaint) in a little water or herb tea.

Wild Chicory Root Tea

Drink two cups of wild chicory root tea* in the course of the day, taking care to sip it slowly. It's a good idea to keep your day's supply in a pre-warmed thermos.

KIDNEYS (damage or injury to)

Agrimony Tea

Drink three cups of agrimony tea* in the course of the day, taking care to sip it slowly.

Calamus Root Tea

Drink one cup of calamus root tea* a day, taking one mouthful before and after each meal. Don't drink more than one cupful in twenty-four hours! It's a good idea to keep your day's supply of tea in a pre-warmed thermos.

Herbal Mixture

Mix equal quantities of golden rod, bedstraw and deadnettles. Drink three or four cups of tea brewed from this mixture in the course of the day. Use one heaping teaspoonful of the mixture for each cup of tea. Pour on hot water and let the herbs steep for thirty seconds before straining them off. It's advisable to continue taking this tea over an extended period.

Knotgrass Tea

Drink two cups of knotgrass tea* in the course of the day, taking care to sip it slowly.

KIDNEYS (stones in)

The following treatments are equally effective for both kidney stones and urinary gravel.

Club Moss Tea

Drink one cup of club moss tea* in the morning before breakfast, taking care to sip it slowly.

Herbal Mixture (1)

Mix equal quantities of bedstraw, deadnettles and golden rod. Drink four cups of tea brewed from this mixture every day; half a cup before breakfast in the morning and the rest in the course of the day, taking small sips at regular intervals. Use one heaping teaspoonful of the mixture for each cup of tea. Pour on hot water and let the herbs steep for thirty seconds before straining them off.

Herbal Mixture (2)

Mix equal quantities (by weight) of birch leaves, restharrow, shepherd's purse and agrimony. Drink two or three cups of tea brewed from this mixture in the course of the day, taking care to sip it slowly.

Use one heaping teaspoonful of the mixture for each cup of tea. Pour on hot water and let the herbs steep for thirty seconds before straining them off.

Horsetail Sitz Baths

A good way of obtaining very speedy relief from both urinary gravel and kidney stones is to drink horsetail tea while taking horsetail sitz baths*. This combination stimulates bladder function, and for the treatment to be effective you should refrain from urinating for as long as you can. This builds up the pressure in the bladder, which helps to wash the gravel and kidney stones out when you finally do go.

The water should be just deep enough to cover your kidneys. Stay in the bath for twenty minutes, and don't dry yourself off when you get out; put on a robe and get straight into bed. Stay there for an hour so that you work up a good sweat.

Drink one to two cups of horsetail tea* while you are taking your sitz bath. Drink the tea slowly, one sip at a time.

Nettle Tea

Drink up to four cups of nettle tea* in the course of the day, taking care to sip it slowly.

Plantain Tea

Drink two to three cups of plantain tea* in the course of the day, taking care to sip it slowly.

You should also take a total of ¼ oz (8g) of plantain seeds a day, washing them down with the plantain tea. This helps to prevent the formation of fresh stones.

LIVER (diseases of)

Agrimony Tea

Drink two cups of agrimony tea* every day as a supplement to the other teas described below, taking care to sip it slowly.

Calamus Root Tea

Drink one mouthful of calamus root tea* before and after each meal, i.e., a total of six mouthfuls a day. This is equivalent to one cup, and it is important not to drink more than this quantity in the course of the day. It's a good idea to keep your day's supply in a pre-warmed thermos.

Calendula Tea

Drink three or four cups of calendula tea* in the course of the day, taking care to sip it slowly.

Celandine Juice

Wash some freshly-picked celandine and run it through a juice extractor without drying it off first. Drink a quarter of a cup of this juice every day, diluted with an equal measure of water.

Dandelion Stems

Eat between five and six raw, freshly-picked dandelion stems every day, washing them carefully beforehand and chewing them very thoroughly. Don't cut off the flowers until after you have washed the plants. The dandelions must be picked while they are in flower.

Herbal Mixture (1)

Mix 2 oz (50g) of speedwell, 2 oz (50g) of dandelion root, 1 oz (25g) of woodruff and 1 oz (25g) of wild chicory flowers. Drink two cups of tea brewed from this mixture every day.

Use one heaping teaspoonful of the mixture for each cup of tea. Pour on hot water and let the herbs steep for thirty seconds before straining them off. Drink the tea slowly, one sip at a time.

Herbal Mixture (2)

Mix 4 oz (100g) of bedstraw, 4 oz (100g) of agrimony and 4 oz (100g) of woodruff. Drink three cups of tea brewed from this mixture every day; the first early in the morning before breakfast.

Use one heaping teaspoonful of the mixture for each cup of tea. Pour on hot water and let the herbs steep for thirty seconds before straining them off. Drink the tea slowly, one sip at a time.

Horsetail Compresses

Relief can be obtained from attacks of liver and gall-bladder disease with the help of these hot horsetail compresses.

Put two generous handfuls of horsetail in a sieve and heat it up over boiling water. When the horsetail is really hot, wrap it up in a clean linen cloth and lay it over your liver, binding it into place with another cloth to keep the heat in. It's best to apply the compress in the evening and to leave it on the whole night long.

Nettle Tea

If you suffer from liver disease it's a very good idea to give yourself a treatment with nettle tea,* drinking four cups a day over a period of several weeks. Drink the tea slowly, one sip at a time.

Plantain Tea

Drink two or three cups of plantain tea* in the course of the day, taking care to sip it slowly.

Sage Tea

Drink up to two cups of sage tea* in the course of the day, taking care to sip it slowly.

Swedish Bitters

Take three tablespoons of Swedish bitters* every day, dissolving each tablespoonful in half a cup of one of the herb teas described in this section. Divide each of these three doses into two portions, taking one of them before eating and the other one afterwards.

Swedish Bitters Compresses

It is also advisable to apply Swedish bitters compresses to the liver. Apply some calendula ointment* before putting the compress on to prevent the alcohol in the bitters from drawing the natural oils out of your skin. Then moisten a suitably large wad of cotton wool with Swedish bitters* and place it over your liver, covering it with a layer of dry cotton wool and a layer of plastic film to keep the warmth in. Bind everything into place with a warm cloth and leave the compress on for four hours.

Wild Chicory Root Tea

Drink two cups of wild chicory root tea* in the course of the day. It's a good idea to keep your day's supply in a pre-warmed thermos.

LIVER (inflammations and infections of)

Dandelion Stems

Eat between five and six raw, freshly-picked dandelion stems every day, washing them carefully beforehand and chewing them very thoroughly. Don't cut off the flowers until after you have washed the plants. The dandelions must be picked while they are in flower.

Ramsons (Broad-leaved Garlic)

The blood-purifying properties of ramsons make it very helpful in treating inflammations and infections of the liver.

Fresh ramsons leaves can be collected in the spring, and should be eaten raw. Wash them, chop them up finely, and sprinkle them on your food as you would fresh parsley. Spinach tastes lovely if you cook it with a few ramsons leaves, and they also make an excellent addition to salads.

Ramsons (Broad-leaved Garlic) Tincture

Drying ramsons destroys its potency, and thus the only way to be able to take advantage of its wonderful healing properties all the year round is to prepare a supply of ramsons tincture.* Take between ten and fifteen drops of ramsons tincture four times a day, dissolved in a little water.

Pathological proliferation of the connective tissue of the liver can also be treated with ramsons.

LUNGS (dilatation of)

Agrimony Tea

Dilatation of the lungs can be cured with agrimony tea.* Drink three cups a day, taking care to sip it slowly.

LUNGS (diseases of)

Calamus Roots

Chewing calamus roots is also helpful. Wash down the bitter juice with a little yarrow tea and spit out the woody residue.

Coltsfoot Syrup

Take a large ceramic or glass container and fill it with alternate layers of freshly-picked and washed coltsfoot leaves and unrefined cane sugar. Give the contents a little time to steep and settle, and then add more layers of coltsfoot leaves and sugar until the container is completely full again. Then seal the mouth with several layers of plastic film, making sure that the seal is completely airtight, and bury the container in a protected spot in the garden. (Take care to cover the mouth of the jar with a piece of wood before you shovel in the earth, otherwise you may make a hole in the plastic film!) In the even, gentle warmth of the earth the sugar and coltsfoot mixture will start to ferment. Dig the container out again after eight weeks and pour the contents into a big cooking pot. Place the pot on the stove and bring the syrup to a gentle boil. Remove it from the heat as soon as it boils, let it cool and then strain it into glass bottles. Take one teaspoonful of this syrup every day, either neat or dissolved in a cup of herb tea.

Horsetail Compresses

Apply a hot horsetail compress to your chest in

the evening before going to sleep and leave it on overnight.

Put two generous handfuls of horsetail in a sieve and heat it up over boiling water. When the horsetail is really hot wrap it up in a clean linen cloth and lay it over your lungs, binding it into place with another cloth to keep the heat in.

Horsetail Tea

Drink two cups of horsetail tea* every day, one before breakfast and the other before your evening meal. Drink the tea slowly, one sip at a time.

Knotgrass Tea

Drink two cups of knotgrass tea* in the course of the day, taking care to sip it slowly.

Nettle Tea

The blood-purifying properties of the nettle make it a useful remedy for diseases of the lungs. Drink two to four cups of nettle tea* in the course of the day, taking care to sip it slowly.

Swedish Bitters Compresses

Apply one Swedish bitters compress to your chest every day, leaving it on for four hours. If you find that it helps, you can apply a second compress to your back at the same time. Apply some calendula ointment* before putting the compress on to prevent the alcohol in the bitters from drawing the natural oils out of your skin. Then moisten a wad of cotton wool with Swedish bitters* and lay it over your lungs, covering it with a layer of dry cotton wool and a layer of plastic foil to keep the heat in. Bind everything into place with a warm cloth.

Yarrow Tea

Drink four cups of yarrow tea* in the course of the day, taking care to sip it slowly.

LUPUS

Lupus is an ulcerative tubercular skin disease that most frequently affects the face.

Horsetail Wash

Lupus can be treated successfully by bathing the affected areas with this horsetail wash.

Pour 1 pt (½ l) of hot water into a bowl containing two heaping teaspoonfuls of horsetail and let it steep for half a minute before straining it and bathing the affected areas with the liquid.

You can also use the strained-off horsetail in warm compresses. Wrap it up in a clean linen cloth and apply it directly to the affected skin, binding it on with another cloth to keep the heat in.

Yarrow Wash

Pour 1 pt (½ l) of hot water into a bowl containing two heaping teaspoonfuls of yarrow and let it steep for half a minute before straining it and bathing the affected areas with the liquid.

LYMPH NODES (dysfunction of)

Bedstraw Tea

Dysfunctions of the lymph nodes can be regulated with the help of bedstraw tea.* Drink two or three cups in the course of the day, taking care to sip it slowly.

LYMPH NODES (lymphadenopathy)

Lymphadenopathy can be treated externally with embrocations and compresses. Calendula ointment is also helpful. If a lymphadenectomy (surgical removal of the lymph nodes) has been carried out, you should apply Swedish bitters compresses and hot horsetail compresses.

Fresh Leaf Dressings

For making these dressings you can use bedstraw leaves, butterbur leaves, plantain leaves, or calendula leaves and stems. Wash the freshly-pickled leaves carefully, crush them to a pulp on a wooden chopping board using a rolling pin and apply the pulp directly to the swollen lymph nodes. Try out the different kinds of leaves in turn until you find the one that agrees with you the best.

Herbal Mixture

Mix 4 oz (100g) of stinging nettles, 4 oz (100g) of yarrow, 12 oz (300g) of calendula and 4 oz (100g) of horsetail. Drink six to eight cups of tea brewed from this mixture every day. Use one heaping teaspoonful of the mixture for each cup of tea. Pour on hot water and let the herbs steep for thirty seconds before straining them off. Drink the tea slowly, one sip at a time.

Marjoram Oil
Gently rub a little marjoram oil* into the swollen lymph nodes.

St John's Wort Oil
Apply a little St John's wort oil* to the swollen lymph nodes several times a day.

Swedish Bitters
Take three tablespoons of Swedish bitters* a day, dissolving each tablespoonful in half a cup of the mixed herb tea, described above. Divide each of these three doses into two portions and take one of them before eating and the other one afterward.

LYMPH NODES (swollen)

St John's Wort Oil
Swollen lymph nodes can be treated effectively with St John's wort oil.* gently massage a little of the oil into the swollen nodes several times a day.

METABOLISM (diseases of)

Calamus Root Tea
Calamus helps to stimulate the metabolism. Drink one mouthful of myrtle flag root tea* before and after each meal, i.e., a total of six mouthfuls a day. This is equivalent to one cup, and it is important not to drink more than this quantity in any one day. It's a good idea to keep your day's supply in a pre-warmed thermos.

Dandelion Stems
Eat ten raw, freshly-picked dandelion stems every day, washing them carefully beforehand and chewing them very thoroughly. Don't cut off the flowers until after you have washed the plants. The dandelions must be picked while they are in flower.

Mistletoe Tea
Drink two or three cups of mistletoe tea* every day (depending on the severity of the disease), taking care to sip it slowly. It's a good idea to keep your day's supply in a pre-warmed thermos.

If you suffer from a metabolic disease it's helpful to give yourself a full course of treatment with mistletoe tea. (See page 120.)

Wild Chicory Tea
Drink one cup of wild chicory tea* every morning, taking care to sip it slowly.

MISCARRIAGES

Hornbeam Sprout Soup
A soup made from the tips of the fresh young leaves of the hornbeam tree can help to prevent miscarriages.

Pour 1 pt (½ l) of milk into a saucepan, add a handful of fresh leaf-tips and bring the mixture to the boil. Strain off the leaves, add an egg yolk and thicken the soup with a simple roux made with oil and flour. Eat a bowlful of this soup every day with your evening meal. (It's perfectly all right to continue with this treatment for several weeks, or even for several months if you like.)

Lady's Mantle Tea
Lady's mantle tea* can also help to prevent miscarriages. You should start taking it at the beginning of the fourth month of pregnancy. Drink four cups every day.

Lady's Mantle and Yarrow Tea
Mix equal quantities of lady's mantle and yarrow. Use one heaping teaspoonful of this mixture for each cup of tea. Pour on hot water and let the herbs steep for thirty seconds before straining them off. Drink two to three cups of this tea in the course of the day, taking care to sip it slowly.

Thyme Tea
Drink two cups of thyme tea* during the day, sipping it slowly.

MULTIPLE SCLEROSIS

This terrible disease is regarded as incurable, and although the medicinal herbs from God's garden *can* help, the process does take time, and one needs to have a great deal of perseverance and faith in the herbs' ability to assist the patient.

Use fresh herbs rather than dried ones if possible, as their potency is greater, and do remember to pick and dry an adequate supply to tide you over the winter months.

Please don't try to use all of the herbs and recipes listed below at the same time! It wouldn't help, and in any case it would be impossible. All you need to know is that all of the teas, bath infusions and tinctures described here *can* help; which ones you use and the order in which you use them is something that you must decide with the help of your own intuition (it will also depend on the availability of the individual herbs).

Chamomile Oil
Massage your entire body with chamomile oil.*

Chamomile Tincture
Fill a glass bottle with freshly-picked chamomile flowers and cover them completely with 38-40% grain alcohol. Leave the sealed bottle to stand in a warm place for at least two weeks. Massage this tincture into the joints, hips and spine.

Comfrey Root Poultices
If the disease causes stiffness of the spine, apply warm comfrey root poultices.

Add a tablespoonful of powdered comfrey root and a few drops of vegetable oil to a cupful of hot water and mix well until the consistency is smooth. Then apply the warm paste to a clean linen cloth and place it directly on the affected part of the spine, binding it gently into place with another cloth.

Comfrey Root Tincture
Gently massage some comfrey root tincture* into the affected parts of the body.

Nettle and Thyme Baths
Soak 8 oz (200g) of either stinging nettles or thyme in 1 gal (5 l) of cold water for twelve hours. Then heat up the infusion gently and strain the liquid into your bathwater. It is important that your heart should not be below the water level. Stay in the bath for twenty minutes, and don't dry yourself off when you get out; put on a robe and get straight into bed. Stay there for an hour so that you work up a good sweat. Alternate between nettle baths and thyme baths, taking one every week.

Sage Tea
Take two cups of sage tea* every day as a supplement to the lady's mantle tea (see below). Drink it slowly, one sip at a time.

St John's Wort Oil
Gently massage the entire body with St John's wort oil*. It's a particularly good idea to rub some into your skin before applying any of the alcohol-based tinctures described here.

St John's Wort Tincture
Massage St John's wort tincture* into the joints, hips and spine.

Sitz Baths
Sitz baths made with infusions of pine needles, St John's wort, chamomile, sage, yarrow, thyme or horsetail are all helpful in the treatment of all kinds of paralysis. One shouldn't try to overdo it however: don't mix the different herbs and don't use more than one kind in any one week.

No matter which of the different herbs you are using the preparation and treatment is always the same. First soak 4 oz (100g) of the herbs in 1 gal (5 l) of cold water for twelve hours. Then heat up the infusion gently and strain the liquid into your bathwater. The water should be just deep enough to cover your kidneys. Stay in the bath for twenty minutes, and don't dry yourself off when you get out; put on a robe and get straight into bed. Stay there for an hour so that you work up a good sweat.

Sorrel Juice
Wash some freshly-picked common sorrel leaves and run them through a juice extractor while they are still wet. Take three to five drops of this juice six times a day at hourly intervals, dissolving it in a little of one of the herb teas described in this section.

Swedish Bitters
Take three tablespoons of Swedish bitters* a day, dissolving each tablespoonful in half a cup of water or herb tea. Divide each of these three doses into two portions, taking one of them before eating and the other one afterwards.

Swedish Bitters Compresses
Apply one Swedish bitters compress to the back of the head every day and leave it on for four hours. Moisten a wad of cotton wool with Swedish bitters* and bind it gently onto the back of your head with a clean cloth or bandage.

Thyme Oil
Fill a glass bottle with freshly-picked thyme flowers and pour in enough oil to cover them completely. Seal the bottle and leave it to stand in a warm place for three weeks. Gently massage this oil into the entire body. It's best to apply one of these herb oils before using any of the tinctures, as the latter are alcohol-based and they tend to deplete the skin's natural oils.

Yarrow Tea

Take two cups of yarrow tea* a day, one in the morning and one in the evening. Drink it slowly, one sip at a time.

Yarrow Tincture

Massage yarrow tincture* into the joints, hips and spine.

If all three of the tinctures described here are available (St John's wort, chamomile and yarrow) it's best to alternate between the three, using a different one each week.

MUSCLES (atrophy of)

Lady's Mantle Tea

Drink four cups of lady's mantle tea* in the course of the day, taking care to sip it slowly. Use freshly-picked lady's mantle if it is at all possible.

Shepherd's Purse Tincture

Massage shepherd's purse tincture* into the affected muscles three times a day.

Thyme Oil

Used as an embrocation, thyme oil* supplements the effects of the shepherd's purse tincture, so it's a good idea to alternate between the tincture and the oil. Massage the oil into the affected muscles several times a day.

MUSCLES (disorders of)

Lady's Mantle and Shepherd's Purse Tea

This tea is a good treatment for muscle disorders. Use one heaping teaspoonful of a mixture made from equal measures of lady's mantle and shepherd's purse for each cup of tea. Pour on hot water and let the herbs steep for thirty seconds before straining them off. Drink two to three cups of the tea in the course of the day, taking care to sip it slowly.

Shepherd's Purse Tincture

Use shepherd's purse tincture* as an embrocation, applying it to the affected muscles several times a day.

MYOMAS

Myomas are benign tumors composed of muscle tissue.

Yarrow Sitz Baths

In my experience yarrow sitz baths* are the only successful treatment available for myomas. Stay in the bath for twenty minutes, and don't dry yourself off when you get out; put on a robe and get straight into bed. Stay there for an hour so that you work up a good sweat.

NERVE INJURIES OR LESIONS

St John's Wort Tea

Drink three cups of St John's wort tea* in the course of the day, taking care to sip it slowly.

NERVOUS DISORDERS

Bedstraw Tea

Drink two to three cups of bedstraw tea* a day, taking care to sip it slowly.

St John's Wort Tea

Drink three cups of St John's wort tea* in the course of the day, taking care to sip it slowly.

Thyme Baths

Soak 6 oz (200g) of thyme in 1 gal (5 l) of cold water for twelve hours. Then heat up the infusion gently and strain the liquid into your bathwater. It is important that your heart should be above the water level. Stay in the bath for twenty minutes, and don't dry yourself off when you get out; put on a robe and get straight into bed. Stay there for an hour so that you work up a good sweat. Take one thyme bath every month for two months.

Thyme Tea

Drink two to three cups of thyme tea* in the course of the day, taking care to sip it slowly.

NEURALGIA

Neuralgia is a condition in which severe spasmodic pains are experienced along one or more nerves.

Chamomile Oil

Used as an embrocation, chamomile oil* is a good treatment for neuralgia. Gently massage the oil into the affected areas.

Horse Chestnut Compresses

Peel some horse chestnuts and grind them up in a blender. Fill a small pillowcase or cushion cover with the ground chestnuts and apply it to the affected area.

NEURITIS

Horse Chestnut Compresses

Peel some fresh horse chestnuts and grind them up in a blender. Stuff a small pillowcase or cushion cover with the ground chestnuts and apply it to the affected area.

Nettles

Neuritis in the arms or legs can be treated by stroking the affected areas very gently with a freshly-picked stinging nettle.

St John's Wort Tea

Drink three cups of St John's wort tea* in the course of the day, taking care to sip it slowly.

Yarrow Wash

Neuritis in the arms or legs can also be treated by bathing the affected areas with warm yarrow wash. Soak 4 oz (100g) of yarrow in 1 gal (5 l) of cold water for twelve hours, and when the time is up heat up the infusion gently and sieve off the yarrow.

NEUROSES

St John's Wort Tincture

You should use St John's wort oil* every day, both externally for massages and also internally, taking between ten and fifteen drops a day dissolved in a little water.

OPERATION WOUNDS

Calendula Ointment

Large operational wounds can be extremely uncomfortable. The tightness and pulling of the skin around them while they are healing can be particularly unpleasant for instance, but this can be alleviated with the help of calendula ointment.* Gently rub a little of the ointment into the affected area several times a day.

Swedish Bitters

The healing of stubborn operational wounds can be speeded up with the help of Swedish bitters.*

Take one tablespoonful three times a day in a little water or herb tea.

PANCREAS (diseases of)

Calamus Root Tea

Drink one mouthful of calamus root tea* before and after each meal, i.e., a total of six mouthfuls a day. This is equivalent to one cup, and it is important not to drink more than this quantity in one day. It's a good idea to keep your day's supply in a pre-warmed thermos.

Calendula Ointment

Calendula ointment should be rubbed into the skin before you apply the Swedish bitters compresses (see below).

Melt 8 oz (250g) of pure lard in a saucepan and add two generous handfuls of calendula leaves, flowers and stems. Proceed according to the standard recipe for calendula ointment.*

Herbal Mixture

Take 4 oz (100g) of stinging nettles, 12 oz (300g) of calendula and 4 oz (100g) of yarrow and mix them well. Drink between 2½ and 3½ pt (1½-2 l) of tea made from this herbal mixture every day. To make 3 pt (1¾ l) of tea take seven heaping teaspoonfuls of the herbal mixture (one teaspoon per cup) and pour on 3 pt (1¾ l) of hot water, letting it steep for thirty seconds before straining off the herbs and transferring the tea to a pre-warmed thermos. Drink the tea slowly, taking one mouthful every twenty minutes. (This ensures that your stomach absorbs the tea as completely as possible.)

You should also take between three teaspoons and three tablespoons (depending on how it agrees with you) of Swedish bitters* every day, dissolving each spoonful in half a cup of the tea. Divide each of these three doses into two portions and take one portion before eating and the other afterwards. Sip it very slowly.

Horsetail Compresses

Apply a hot horsetail compress to your stomach twice a day, leaving each compress on for at least two hours. To prepare the compress put two generous handfuls of horsetail in a sieve and heat it up over a pot of boiling water. When its piping hot wrap it up in a clean linen cloth and apply it to your stomach, covering it with a thick warm towel or cloth. Wrap up warm and get into bed, staying there until it's time to remove the compress.

If you wish, you can also apply the compress in the evening and leave it on overnight.

Mistletoe Tea
Drink two cups of mistletoe tea* every day, taking care to sip it slowly. It's a good idea to keep your day's supply in a pre-warmed thermos.

Swedish Bitters
Take three teaspoons of Swedish bitters* a day, dissolving each teaspoonful in half a cup of water or one of the above-mentioned herb teas. Divide each of these three doses into two portions, taking one before eating and one afterward.

Swedish Bitters Compresses
Large Swedish bitters compresses covering the entire abdominal wall can be a very effective treatment for disorders of the pancreas.

Rub the entire area with calendula ointment before you put the compress on so that the alcohol in the bitters doesn't draw the natural oils out of your skin. Then moisten a large wad of cotton wool with Swedish bitters* and tease the cotton wool apart gently so that it covers your entire abdomen, making it as thin as possible. Cover the moist cotton wool with a layer of dry cotton wool to keep the warmth in, and a layer of plastic film to protect your clothes, and bind everything gently into place with a warm cloth. Leave the compress on for four hours. When you take it off, dust your skin with talcum powder to prevent irritation.

PARALYSIS

Sage Tea
Drink two or three cups of sage tea* in the course of the day, taking care to sip it slowly.

Thyme Yea
Drink a cup of thyme tea* in the morning instead of coffee or black tea.

Swedish Bitters
Take three tablespoons of Swedish bitters* every day, dissolving each tablespoonful in half a cup of one of the herb teas mentioned above. Divide each of these three doses into two portions, taking one of them before eating and the other one afterward.

PARALYSIS (of the limbs)

Chamomile Oil
Used as an embrocation, chamomile oil* can help to bring about an improvement. Rub a little of this oil into the affected limbs at regular intervals.

Comfrey Root Poultices
Mix a tablespoonful of powdered comfrey root and a few drops of vegetable oil to a smooth paste with a cupful of hot water. Apply this paste to a clean linen cloth and wrap it around the affected limb, binding it gently into place with another warm cloth.

PARKINSON'S DISEASE

Sorrel Juice
Wash some freshly-picked common sorrel leaves and run them through a juice extractor. Take three to five drops of this juice every hour, diluting it with three parts of herb tea. It's also a good idea to massage the spine with sorrel juice.

Swedish Bitters Compresses
Moisten a wad of cotton wool with Swedish bitters* and apply it to the back of the head. Bind the compress gently into place and leave it on for four hours.

Thyme Baths
A thyme bath can be helpful in cases where the shaking palsy is accompanied by stiffness of the limbs.

Soak 8 oz (200g) of thyme in 1 gal (5 l) of cold water for twelve hours. Then heat up the infusion gently and strain the liquid into your bathwater. It is important that your heart should not be below the water level. Stay in the bath for twenty minutes, and don't dry yourself off when you get out; put on a dressing gown and get straight into bed, staying there for an hour so that you work up a good sweat. Don't take thyme baths very often.

Yarrow Tea
Drink four or five cups of yarrow tea* in the course of the day, taking care to sip it slowly.

Yarrow Tincture
It's advisable to give the spine a gentle massage with an embrocation once a day, alternating sorrel juice and yarrow tincture.*

PERIOSTITIS

Comfrey Root Poultices

The only way of obtaining relief from periostitis — a nasty disease that can be extremely painful — is with hot comfrey root poultices.

Add a tablespoonful of powdered comfrey root and a few drops of vegetable oil to a cup of hot water and mix them well until the consistency is smooth. Apply the warm paste directly to a clean linen cloth and wrap the cloth around the affected area, binding it into place with a second cloth (this should be as thick as possible to keep the heat in). Apply a fresh poultice as soon as the first one cools.

PHANTOM LIMB PAINS

Comfrey Root Poultices

Take a tablespoonful of powdered comfrey root, add a cupful of hot water and a few drops of vegetable oil, and stir the mixture well until smooth. Apply this paste to a clean linen cloth while it is still warm and lay the cloth on the amputation stump. Apply a fresh poultice as soon as the paste becomes cool.

Iris Root Tea

Iris roots should be collected in autumn, because that is when they are at their best. Wash them thoroughly under running water with a brush and then hang them up to dry. When they are completely dry reduce them to a powder in a coffee grinder.

Soak one teaspoonful of this powder in 1 pt (½ l) of cold water for twelve hours, then heat the infusion up gently and strain it. Make the tea last the whole day, taking small sips at regular intervals. It's a good idea to keep it in a pre-warmed thermos.

Onion Tincture

Onion tincture is also helpful for dealing with troublesome phantom limb pains. You can buy it in health food and herbalists' shops, but it can also be made at home very easily.

Fill a glass bottle with freshly-cut onion rings and add enough 38-40% grain alcohol to cover them completely. Leave the sealed bottle to stand in a warm place for at least two weeks. Apply this onion tincture directly to the amputation stump several times a day.

Thyme Baths

Soak a generous handful of thyme in 1 gal (5 l) of cold water for twelve hours, then heat up the infusion gently and strain it into your bathwater. Bathe the stump for twenty minutes, repeating the process three times a week.

Thyme and Club Moss Compresses

Fill a pillowcase with equal quantities of thyme and club moss — 3 to 5 oz (100-150g) of each — heat it up gently in the oven and apply it to the amputation stump, leaving it on overnight.

PHLEBITIS

Calendula Ointment

Calendula ointment* helps to bring relief from phlebitis. Simply apply a little of the ointment to the affected areas.

Coltsfoot Compresses

Wash some freshly-picked coltsfoot leaves and crush them to a pulp on a wooden chopping board using a rolling pin. Mix this pulp with some fresh dairy cream and apply it directly to the infected veins, binding it gently into place with a clean cloth.

Mallow Wash

Bathe your arms and legs in a mallow wash* for twenty minutes.

Swedish Bitters Compresses

After applying calendula ointment* to the affected areas it is also helpful to put on a Swedish bitters compress and to leave it on for four hours.

Moisten a wad of cotton wool with Swedish bitters* and place it over the affected area, covering it with a layer of dry cotton wool and a layer of plastic film to keep the warmth in, and bind everything gently into place with a clean cloth.

PLEURISY

Coltsfoot Tea

Drink two to four cups of coltsfoot tea* a day, taking care to sip it slowly.

Comfrey Root Tea

Drink two to four cups of comfrey root tea* in the course of the day, taking care to sip it slowly.

PNEUMONIA

Plantain and Thyme Tea

Drink plantain and thyme tea* as hot as possible,

taking care to sip it slowly. If an acute case of pneumonia seems to be developing you should drink one cup of this tea every hour. Make each cup of tea fresh just before you drink it.

PROSTATE GLAND (diseases of)

Willow-herb Tea
The small-flowered willow-herb is an effective treatment for all kinds of prostate gland complaints, from simple inflammations to infections. Take two cups of willow-herb tea* in the course of the day, one in the morning before breakfast and the other in the evening before supper. Drink the tea slowly, one sip at a time.

RICKETS

Walnut Leaf Baths
Soak 4 oz (100g) of walnut leaves in 1 gal (5 l) of cold water for twelve hours. Then heat up the infusion gently and strain the liquid into your bathwater. It is important that your heart should not be below the water level. Stay in the bath for twenty minutes, and don't dry yourself off when you get out; put on a robe and get straight into bed. Stay there for an hour so that you work up a good sweat.

SCIATICA

Bracken Compresses
Before going to sleep at night cover the affected area with fresh bracken leaves (take them off the stalks) and bind them into place with a large warm towel. Leave the compress on overnight.

Meadowsweet Tea
Drink two or three cups of meadowsweet tea* in the course of the day, taking care to sip it slowly.

Nettle Baths
Stinging nettle baths are a very effective remedy for sciatica pains.

Soak 8 oz (200g) of stinging nettles in 1 gal (5 l) of cold water for twelve hours. Then heat up the infusion gently and strain the liquid into your bathwater. It's important that your heart should not be below the water level. Stay in the bath for twenty minutes, and don't dry yourself off when you get

out; put on a robe and get straight into bed. Stay there for an hour so that you work up a good sweat.

Sciatica pains in the arms and legs can be treated with fresh nettles. Stroke the affected areas four times with a freshly-picked stinging nettle, starting at the bottom and working upwards. Do this very very gently, and dust the reddened skin with a little talcum powder when you have finished. You should start to feel an improvement after a few days of this treatment.

St John's Wort Oil
Applied as an embrocation, St John's wort oil* brings speedy relief from sciatica. Gently massage the oil into the affected areas.

SHINGLES (herpes zoster)

Herbal Mixture
Mix 1¼ oz (25g) of oak bark, ½ oz (10g) of ladys mantle, 1 oz (20g) of oats, ½ oz (10g) of chamomile, 1¼ oz (25g) of sage and ½ oz (10g) of sweet clover. Put four heaping teaspoonsful of this mixture in 2 pt (1 l) of cold water and heat it up gently until it is just about to come to the boil. Then remove the pot from the heat and let the herbs steep for five minutes before straining them off. Apply a little of the liquid to the affected areas several times a day, dabbing it on very gently with a wad of cotton wool.

You can also use the strained-off herbs in hot compresses. Heat them up gently, wrap them up in a clean linen cloth and apply them directly to the affected area, binding the compress gently into place with another warm cloth. It's best to apply these compresses in the evening and to leave them on overnight.

Houseleek Juice
Wash some freshly-picked houseleek leaves and run them through a juice extractor. Apply the juice to the affected areas several times a day.

SHOCK

Golden Rod Tea
Irritation, stress, worries and sorrow all place a great strain on the kidneys. Golden rod is a particularly good remedy, as it has a very soothing, healing effect on the kidneys. Drink two or three cups of golden rod tea* a day, taking care to sip it slowly.

SHORTNESS OF BREATH

Butterbur Root Tea
Use a level teaspoonful of finely-chopped butterbur root for each cup of tea and soak it in the cold water for twelve hours. Then heat the infusion up gently and strain it. Depending on the severity of the condition, you can drink one or two cups of this tea a day, being sure to sip it slowly.

Calendula Ointment
This calendula ointment should be rubbed into the skin before you apply the Swedish bitters compresses (see below).

Melt 8 oz (250g) of pure lard in a saucepan and add two generous handfuls of calendula leaves, flowers and stems. Proceed according to the standard recipe for calendula ointment.*

Club Moss Tea
Cirrhosis of the liver often causes severe shortness of breath, and this makes it difficult to sleep at night. In cases like this, club moss tea* can work wonders. Drink one cup in the morning before breakfast, taking care to sip it slowly. A second cup may be taken only if you have an extremely serious liver disease, or advanced cirrhosis. In all other cases it's very important not to drink more than the one cupful!

Coltsfoot Inhalations
Coltsfoot vapor inhalations can be very helpful in dealing with attacks of suffocation and choking. Pour some hot water into a bowl containing a heaping tablespoonful of coltsfoot leaves and flowers, cover your head head with a towel and inhale the vapors from the bowl. Repeat this process several times a day.

Horsetail Compresses
A hot horsetail compress placed on the liver and left there overnight can also have very positive effects.

Place a generous handful of horsetail in a sieve and heat it up over boiling water. When it's piping hot, wrap the horsetail in a linen cloth and place it over your liver, covering it with a thick towel to keep in the heat and binding everything into place with a second clean linen cloth.

Mistletoe Tea
If the shortness of breath is a symptom of the menopause, it's advisable to drink one or two cups of mistletoe tea* for quite a long time. Take care to drink the tea slowly, one sip at a time. It's a good idea to keep your day's supply in a pre-warmed thermos.

Ramsons (Broad-leaved Garlic) Wine
Congestion of the lungs often causes breathing difficulties, which can sometimes be really extreme. Ramsons wine* acts as an expectorant, clearing up the congestion and making breathing easier. Let the wine cool before you drink it and make it last the whole day, taking little sips at regular intervals.

Swedish Bitters Compresses
As mentioned above, shortness of breath is often caused by liver disorders. Swedish bitters* compresses help to reduce the pressure on the other organs, such as the bronchi, lungs and heart. The compress should be placed over the liver during the day and left there for four hours. Apply some of the calendula ointment before putting the compress on so that the alcohol in the Swedish bitters doesn't draw the natural oils out of the skin. Then moisten a wad of cotton wool with the bitters and lay it over your liver, covering it with a dry wad of cotton wool to keep in the warmth and a layer of plastic film to protect your clothes, then bind everything into place with another cloth. Dust your skin with a little talcum powder when you remove the compress to prevent any skin irritation.

SKIN DISEASES

Slow-healing skin diseases in which the skin breaks open and begins to weep or suppurate can be treated with a whole series of remedies.

Horsetail and Mallow Washes
First of all, the sores should be bathed very thoroughly with horsetail and mallow washes. Use the horsetail wash first and then the mallow one.

To make the horsetail wash, pour 1 pt (½ l) of hot water into a bowl containing two heaping teaspoonfuls of horsetail and let it steep for thirty seconds before straining it off. Let the wash cool for a while before using it.

For the mallow wash, soak two heaping teaspoonfuls of mallow in 1 pt (½ l) of cold water for twelve hours. Then heat up the infusion gently and strain it. Again, let it cool a little before using it.

Calendula Ointment

Melt 8 oz (250g) of pure lard in a saucepan and add four generous handfuls of finely-chopped calendula leaves, flowers and stems. Proceed according to the standard recipe for calendula ointment.*

Celandine Juice

Then apply a little fresh celandine juice around the edges of the sores. To make the juice, wash some celandine leaves, stems and blossoms and run them through a juice extractor while they are still wet. Apply some calendula ointment around the edges of the sores as soon as the celandine juice has soaked into the skin.

Plantain Leaf Dressings

The open sores themselves should be treated with a dressing made from fresh plantain leaves. Wash some freshly-picked leaves and crush them to a pulp on a wooden chopping board using a rolling pin. Apply the pulp directly to the sores, very gently. If it feels too uncomfortable, rinse the sores out with boiled water and bathe them with the horsetail and mallow washes again. Repeat this process again and again until the plantain leaf pulp feels comfortable on the sores.

You can also use the horsetail and mallow washes described above in compresses. Before going to bed at night soak a clean cloth in one of the warm washes and wrap it around the sores, binding it gently into place with another warm cloth. Leave the compress on the whole night long.

If the sores are very large or if they are in a number of different places all over your body, apply some fresh plantain or great plantain leaf pulp to a large linen cloth and wrap it around your entire body when you go to bed in the evening, leaving it on overnight.

Horsetail and Mallow Baths

If the sores are large, it is best to take horsetail and mallow baths instead of bathing them with the washes. For each bath, soak 8 oz (200g) of horsetail or mallow in 1 gal (5 l) of cold water for twelve hours, and then heat up this infusion gently and strain the liquid into your bathwater. It's important that your heart should not be below the water level. Stay in the bath for twenty minutes, and don't dry yourself off when you get out; put on a robe and get straight into bed. Stay there for an hour so that you work up a good sweat.

Thyme Baths

Thyme baths also help to speed up the healing of this kind of skin disease.

Soak 8 oz (200g) of thyme in 1 gal (5 l) of cold water for twelve hours. Then heat up the infusion gently and sieve off the thyme. It's important that your heart should not be below the water level. Stay in the bath for twenty minutes, and don't dry yourself off when you get out; put on a robe and get straight into bed. Stay there for an hour so that you work up a good sweat.

Herbal Mixture (1)

Mix equal quantities of stinging nettles, speedwell, calendula and yarrow. Take four cups of tea brewed from this mixture every day (in addition to the external treatments described above), to help purify your blood. Use one heaping teaspoonful of this mixture for each cup of tea. Pour on hot water and let the herbs steep for thirty seconds before straining them off. Drink the tea slowly, one sip at a time.

Herbal Mixture (2)

The healing of the sores can be speeded up with the help of a tea made from stinging nettles, calendula and yarrow. Mix 4 oz (100g) of stinging nettles with 12 oz (300g) of calendula and 4 oz (100g) of yarrow, then prepare the tea following the method described for the first herbal mixture. Drink four cups of this tea daily, taking care to sip it slowly.

SKIN DISEASES (chronic)

Bedstraw Juice

Wash some freshly-picked bedstraw and run it through a juice extractor. Apply some of this juice directly to the affected areas several times a day.

Ramsons (Broad-leaved Garlic)

The blood-purifying properties of ramsons make it very useful in the treatment of chronic skin diseases.

Fresh ramsons leaves can be collected in the spring and should be eaten raw. Wash the leaves, chop them up finely, and sprinkle them on your food as you would fresh parsley. Spinach tastes lovely if you cook it with a few ramsons leaves, and they also make an excellent addition to salads.

Speedwell and Nettle Tea

If you suffer from a chronic skin disease, you should drink two cups of this tea every day. Mix equal parts of speedwell and fresh stinging nettle leaf-tips and use one heaping teaspoonful of this mixture for each cup of tea. Pour on hot water and let the herbs steep for thirty seconds before straining them off. Drink the tea slowly, one sip at a time.

SPEECH DISORDERS

St John's Wort Sitz Baths and Footbaths
Soak 4 oz (100g) of St John's wort in 1 gal (5 l) of cold water for twelve hours. Then heat up the infusion gently and strain the liquid into your bathwater. The water should be just deep enough to cover your kidneys. Stay in the bath for twenty minutes, and don't dry yourself off when you get out; put on a robe and get straight into bed. Stay there for an hour so that you work up a good sweat.

Take a St John's wort sitz bath on three days of the week, and St John's wort footbaths on the other four days. Prepare the infusion for the footbaths in exactly the same way as described above, but using half the quantity of St John's wort.

St John's Wort Tea
Drink two or three cups of St John's wort tea* in the course of the day, taking care to sip it slowly.

Swedish Bitters Compresses
Speech defects and stuttering can be treated effectively with the help of daily Swedish bitters compresses applied to the back of the head. Moisten a wad of cotton wool with Swedish bitters* and place it on the back of your head, binding it gently into place with a clean cloth. Leave the compress on for four hours.

SPHINCTER (weakness of)

Calamus Root Tea
Drink one mouthful of calamus root tea* before and after each meal, i.e., a total of six mouthfuls a day. This is equivalent to one cup, and it is important not to drink more than this quantity in the course of the day. It's a good idea to keep your day's supply in a pre-warmed thermos.

Lady's Mantle Tea
Drink four cups of lady's mantle tea* in the course of the day, taking care to sip it slowly.

Shepherd's Purse Tincture
Gently massage a little shepherd's purse tincture* into the anus several times a day, and take ten drops internally three times a day in a little lady's mantle tea.

Swedish Bitters Compresses
If the shepherd's purse tincture is not available immediately, you can apply Swedish bitters compresses instead. Moisten a small wad of cotton wool with Swedish bitters* and apply it directly to the anus.

SPINE (injuries)

Bedstraw Ointment
This bedstraw ointment is very helpful for treating spinal injuries. Massage it gently into the spine once a day, starting at the bottom and working upwards.

To make the ointment, first melt 8 oz (250g) of pure lard in a saucepan and then add a generous handful of bedstraw flowers. Proceed according to the standard recipe for ointment.*

Yarrow Tincture
To supplement the effects of the bedstraw ointment, massage a little yarrow tincture* into the spine once a day.

Thyme and Yarrow Baths
In addition to the treatments described above it's a good idea to take daily hot baths with infusions of thyme or yarrow, alternating the two.

Soak 8 oz (200g) of thyme or yarrow in 1 gal (5 l) of cold water for twelve hours. Then heat up the infusion gently and strain the liquid into your bathwater. It is important that your heart should not be below the water level. Stay in the bath for twenty minutes, and don't dry yourself off when you get out; put on a dressing gown and get straight into bed, staying there for an hour so that you work up a good sweat.

SPLEEN (diseases of)

Agrimony Tea
Drink two cups of agrimony tea* in the course of the day, taking care to sip it slowly.

Calamus Root Tea
Drink one mouthful of calamus root tea* before

and after each meal, i.e., a total of six mouthfuls a day. This is equivalent to one cup, and it is important not to drink more than this quantity in any one day.

Dandelion Stems

Eat between four and six raw, freshly-picked dandelion stems every day, washing them carefully beforehand and chewing them very thoroughly. Don't cut off the flowers until after you have washed the plants. The dandelions must be picked while they are in flower.

Herbal Mixture

Mix 2 oz (50g) of speedwell, 2 oz (50g) of dandelion root, 1 oz (25g) of woodruff and 1 oz (25g) of wild chicory flowers. Drink two cups of tea brewed from this mixture in the course of the day. Use one heaped teaspoonful of the mixture for each cup of tea. Pour on hot water and let the herbs steep for thirty seconds before straining them off. Drink the tea slowly, one sip at a time.

Nettle Tea

The blood-purifying properties of the nettle make it a good choice for the treatment of diseases of the spleen. Drink up to four cups of nettle tea* in the course of the day, taking care to sip it slowly.

Wild Chicory Root Tea

Drink two cups of wild chicory root tea* in the course of the day, taking care to sip it slowly. It's a good idea to keep your day's supply in a pre-warmed thermos.

STOMACH (gastric acid)

Calamus Root Tea

Calamus roots helps to normalize the production of gastric acid, no matter whether your stomach is producing too much or too little.

Drink one mouthful of calamus root tea* before and after each meal, i.e., a total of six mouthfuls a day. This is equivalent to one cup, and it is important not to drink more than this quantity in any one day. It's a good idea to keep your day's supply in a pre-warmed thermos.

STOMACH (gastric ulcers)

Calendula Tea

Drink two to three cups of calendula tea* in the course of the day, taking care to sip it slowly.

Herbal Mixture

Mix 4 oz (100g) of comfrey, 2 oz (50g) of calendula and 2 oz (50g) of knotgrass. Drink two to four cups of tea brewed from this mixture a day. Use one heaping teaspoonful of the mixture for each cup of tea. Pour on hot water and let the herbs steep for thirty seconds before straining them off. Drink the tea slowly, one sip at a time.

Knotgrass Tea

Drink two cups of knotgrass tea* in the course of the day, taking care to sip it slowly.

Mallow Leaves

Another good remedy for gastric ulcers is a barley soup garnished with freshly-pickled mallow leaves. First prepare the barley soup and let it cool before you add the mallow leaves. Then wash the mallow leaves, chop them up finely and sprinkle them in the soup.

Nettle Tea

Drink up to four cups of nettle tea* a day, taking care to sip it slowly. Stinging nettle tea is the ideal choice for an extended course of treatment as it is perfectly all right to drink it every day over a period of several weeks.

STROKES

Fortunately there are a number of symptoms that can help us to predict an impending stroke, making it possible to take preventive steps in good time — God's garden provides us with a number of good preventive remedies. These symptoms include feelings of giddiness, feelings of fear with no apparent reason, intense restlessness and auditory hallucinations (hearing nonexistent voices, for instance).

PREVENTIVE REMEDIES

Of course, the first thing to do is to consult a doctor without delay. It is also very important to eliminate alcohol, nicotine and caffeine from your diet completely. Eat a moderate amount of good, nutritious food and be sure to get plenty of fresh air.

Herbal Mixture

Mix equal quantities of angelica root, lamb's quarters, pyrethrum, cinquefoil, lavender blossoms, marjoram, masterwort, avens, rosemary, sage, sweet violets, and hyssop. Drink several cups of tea brewed from this mixture every day, making each cup fresh just before you drink it. This tea must be made with apple juice instead of water, and it is important to use organically-produced additive-free juice. Use a heaping teaspoonful of the mixture for each cup of tea, pour on the hot apple juice and let the herbs steep for thirty seconds before straining them off. Drink the tea slowly, one sip at a time.

Mistletoe Tea
Drink two cups of mistletoe tea* every day — one in the morning and the other in the evening — taking care to sip it slowly. It's a good idea to keep your day's supply in a pre-warmed thermos.

Sage Tea
Drink two cups of sage tea every day, taking care to sip it slowly.

Swedish Bitters Compresses
It's advisable to apply one Swedish bitters compress to the kidneys every day. Apply some calendula ointment* before you put on the compress to prevent the alcohol in the Swedish bitters from drawing the natural oils out of your skin. Then moisten a wad of cotton wool with Swedish bitters* and place it over your kidneys, covering it with a layer of dry cotton wool and a layer of plastic film to keep the warmth in. Bind everything gently into place with a warm cloth and leave the compress on for four hours. These compresses should be applied during the daytime.

Cold compresses on the heart are also helpful. Soak a clean cloth in cold water, wring it out and apply it to your heart as a compress.

TREATMENT
There is no reason to lose heart after having a stroke — there are medicinal herbs in God's garden that can be of help even in cases involving partial paralysis.

Mistletoe Tea
It's a good idea to start a six-week treatment with mistletoe tea.* Drink three cups a day in the first three weeks, two cups a day in the next two weeks and one cup a day during the last week. Drink the tea slowly, one sip at a time. Keep your day's supply in a pre-warmed thermos otherwise you will have to heat the tea up in a hot water bath before drinking it.

Baths
Take one bath with an infusion of yarrow, horsetail or thyme every week. Take a yarrow sitz bath the first week, a horsetail sitz bath the second week,

a full thyme bath (i.e., not a sitz bath) the third week, and then begin again with the yarrow the week after that.

To prepare the infusions, take 4 oz (100g) of horsetail or yarrow (for the sitz baths) or 8 oz (200g) of thyme (for a full bath) and soak it in 1 gal (5 l) of cold water for twelve hours. Then heat up the infusion gently and strain the liquid into your bathwater. The water in the sitz baths should be just deep enough to cover your kidneys; the water in the full bath will be deeper of course, but it is important that your heart should not be below the water level. Stay in the bath for twenty minutes, and don't dry yourself off when you get out; put on a robe and get straight into bed. Stay there for an hour so that you work up a good sweat.

Comfrey Compresses
Wash some freshly-picked comfrey leaves and place them in a bowl. Pour on hot water and let the leaves steep for a few moments until they are really hot. Then strain them off, wrap them in a clean linen cloth and apply them directly to the paralysed area.

Another pleasant way of obtaining relief is to fill a pillowcase or cushion cover with dried bracken leaves (remove the stems first) and to place it under your head at night instead of your pillow.

Embrocations
The parts of the body that have become paralysed as the result of a stroke should be massaged with a tincture made from shepherd's purse,* St John's wort*, yarrow* or thyme* several times a day.

Supplement the effects of the tincture with either thyme oil* or St John's wort oil.* Gently massage one of these oils into the affected areas several times a day.

Herbal Mixture
Mix equal quantities of speedwell, St John's wort, lavender, lemon balm, rosemary and sage. Drink two cups of tea brewed from this mixture every day — one in the morning and the other in the afternoon. Use one heaping teaspoonful of the mixture for each cup of tea. Pour on hot water and let the herbs steep for thirty seconds before straining them off. Drink the tea slowly, one sip at a time.

Swedish Bitters Compresses
It's advisable to apply one Swedish bitters

compress to the back of the head every day; this promotes the circulation of blood in the brain. Moisten a wad of cotton wool with Swedish bitters* and place it over the back of the head, binding it gently into place with a cloth. Leave the compress on for two hours.

STUTTERING

See Speech Defects.

THROMBOSIS

Nettle Footbaths
Once a thrombosis has cleared up it's a good idea to take nettle footbaths to improve the circulation, but please do have your doctor confirm that the thrombosis *has* cleared before you start taking the footbaths.

Soak either two generous handfuls of fresh stinging nettles (this is preferable) or 4 oz (100g) of dried nettles in 1 gal (25 l) of cold water for twelve hours. Then heat up the infusion gently and bathe your feet in it for twenty minutes without removing the nettles.

Plantain Dressings
Wash some freshly-picked plantain leaves, crush them to a pulp on a wooden chopping board using a rolling pin and apply the pulp directly to the affected area.

Swedish Bitters Compresses
Apply some calendula ointment* before you put the compress on to prevent the alcohol in the bitters from drawing the natural oils out of your skin. Then moisten a wad of cotton wool with Swedish bitters* and place it over the affected area, covering it with a layer of dry cotton wool and a layer of plastic film to keep the warmth in, then bind everything gently into place with a warm cloth.

TREMORS

Herbal Mixture
Mix equal quantities (by weight) of ash leaves, St John's wort flowers, yarrow, sage and horsetail. Drink three cups of tea brewed from this mixture during the day.

Use one heaping teaspoonful of the mixture for each cup of tea. Pour on hot water and let the herbs steep for thirty seconds before straining them off. Drink the tea slowly, one sip at a time.

Herbal Tincture
Take 2½ oz (50g) of St John's wort, 1 oz (20g) of orchis, 1 oz (20g) of cowslips and ½ oz (10g) of juniper berries and put them in a glass bottle. Then add enough 38-40% grain alcohol to cover them completely, seal the bottle and leave it to stand in a warm place for at least two weeks. Take between ten and fifteen drops of this tincture every hour in a little of the mixed herb tea described above.

Sitz Baths
These herbal sitz baths should be taken in a three-week cycle. Take three sitz baths in the first week and then take a two-week break, followed by another three sitz baths in the next week and another two-week break, and so on. Don't use more than one variety of herb for preparing the bath infusion in any one week. Pine needles, St John's wort, yarrow and thyme are all suitable for these baths. Do use fresh herbs if you possibly can, as they are more potent than the dried variety.

To prepare one bath first soak 4 oz (100g) (dried) or half a bucketful (fresh) of herbs in 1 gal (5 l) of cold water for twelve hours. Then heat the infusion up gently and strain the liquid into your bathwater. The water should be just deep enough to cover your kidneys. Stay in the bath for twenty minutes, and don't dry yourself off when you get out; put on a robe and get straight into bed. Stay there for an hour so that you work up a good sweat.

TRIGEMINAL NEURALGIA (tic douleureux)

Herbal Mixture
Mix equal quantities of St John's wort, chamomile, mullein, yarrow and thyme flowers and add one measure of club moss spores. Drink four cups of tea brewed from this mixture in the course of the day. Use one heaping teaspoonful of the mixture for each cup of tea. Pour on hot water and let the herbs steep for thirty seconds before straining them off.

You can also fill a small pillowcase or cushion cover with the mixture and apply it to the affected area as a compress.

Horse Chestnut Compresses

Another good way of obtaining relief from trigeminal (or facial) neuralgia is to apply a horse chestnut compress. Peel enough fresh horse chestnuts to fill a small pillowcase or cushion cover and grind them up in a blender. Sew them up in the pillowcase and apply it to the affected area as a compress. Alternatively, you can fill the pillowcase with finely-chopped club moss.

Nettle Wash

If you are in pain, it's helpful to bathe your face with this wash made from stinging nettles.

Pour 1 pt (½ l) of hot water into a bowl containing a handful of stinging nettles and let them steep for thirty seconds before straining them off. Bathe your face thoroughly with the liquid. When you have finished, dry your skin gently with a towel and apply a small linen bag filled with club moss.

St John's Wort Oil

St John's wort oil* makes a good embrocation for painful facial neuralgia. Gently massage this oil into the affected areas several times a day.

Swedish Bitters

Take three teaspoons of Swedish bitters* every day. Dissolve each teaspoonful in half a cup of the mixed herb tea (see above) and divide each of these three doses into two portions, taking one before eating and the other one afterward.

Swedish Bitters Compresses

Swedish bitters compresses are another good external remedy. Apply some calendula ointment* before putting the compress on so that the alcohol in the bitters doesn't draw the natural oils out of your skin. Then moisten a wad of cotton wool with Swedish bitters and lay it on the affected area, covering it with a layer of dry cotton wool and a layer of plastic film to keep the warmth in and binding everything gently into place with a warm cloth. It's best to go to bed while the compress is doing its work, leaving it on for between two and four hours.

ULCERS

Bedstraw Tea

Mouth ulcers can be treated by gargling and rinsing out the mouth with warm bedstraw tea.* Gargle with the tea several times a day.

Butterbur Dressings

Wash some freshly-picked butterbur leaves and crush them to a pulp on a wooden chopping board using a rolling pin. Apply this pulp directly to the ulcer. The dressing must be changed several times a day.

Calendula Tincture Dressings

Soak a clean linen cloth in calendula tincture* diluted with an equal quantity of boiled water and apply it to the affected area.

Celandine Juice

Wash some freshly-picked celandine leaves, blossoms and stems and run them through a juice extractor without drying them off first. Apply a little of this juice to the affected area several time a day with a small wad of cotton wool.

Drink a quarter of a cup of the celandine juice every day, diluting it with an equal quantity of water.

Coltsfoot Dressings

These coltsfoot dressings are a good treatment for scrofulous ulcers.

Use two heaping teaspoons of coltsfoot for each cup of water. Pour on the hot water and let the herbs steep for thirty seconds before straining them off. Soak a clean cloth in the warm liquid and apply it to the affected area, binding it gently into place with a thick cloth to keep in the warmth.

Apply some calendula ointment* before you put the compress on in order to prevent the alcohol in the bitters from drawing the natural oils out of your skin. Then moisten a wad of cotton wool with Swedish bitters and apply it to the affected area, covering it with a layer of dry cotton wool to keep the warmth in and a layer of plastic film to protect your clothing. Bind everything into place with a warm cloth and leave the compress on for four hours.

Deadnettle Dressings

Pour 1 pt (½ l) of hot water into a bowl containing three heaped teaspoonfuls of deadnettles and let them steep for half a minutes before straining the infusion. Soak a clean cloth in this liquid and apply it to the ulcer, binding it gently into place with a thick cloth to keep it warm.

Horsetail Poultices

Put two heaping handfuls of horsetail in a sieve and heat it up over boiling water. When the horsetail is really hot, wrap it up in a clean linen cloth and apply it to the affected area, binding it gently into place with a thick cloth to keep in the warmth. Leave the poultice on for several hours.

Horsetail Tea
Drink two or three cups of horsetail tea* in the course of the day, taking care to sip it slowly.

Lady's Mantle Tea
Drink two or three cups of lady's mantle tea* in the course of the day, taking care to sip it slowly.

Mallow Wash
Soak the affected areas in a mallow wash* for twenty minutes. (Alternatively you can simply rinse the ulcers out with the wash. This must be repeated several times.)

Sorrel Juice
Fresh sorrel juice helps both internal and external ulcers to heal better.

Wash some freshly-picked common sorrel leaves and run them through a juice extractor. Take between three and five drops of this juice every hour in a little water or herb tea.

If the ulcers are external apply a little freshly-pressed sorrel juice to them directly several times a day.

Swedish Bitters Compresses
In addition to the hot horsetail poultices it is also advisable to apply Swedish bitters* compresses as they are very effective for the treatment of all kinds of ulcers.

Instead of bedstraw tea you can also gargle with myrrh tincture. Dissolve between thirty and forty drops of the tincture in a cup of lukewarm water.

URINARY GRAVEL

Herbal Mixture
Make a mixture of equal measures (by weight) of birch leaves, restharrow, shepherd's purse and agrimony. Drink two cups of tea made from this mixture every day, using one heaping teaspoonful of the herbs for each cup of tea. Pour on hot water and let the herbs steep for thirty seconds before straining them off. Drink the tea slowly, one sip at a time.

Horsetail Sitz Baths
A good way of obtaining very speedy relief from urinary gravel is to drink horsetail tea while taking a horsetail sitz bath.* This combination stimulates the functioning of the bladder, and for the treatment to be effective you should refrain from urinating for as long as you can. This builds up the pressure in the bladder, which helps to wash the gravel out of your urinary tract when you eventually empty your bladder.

Stay in the bath for twenty minutes, and don't dry yourself off when you get out; put on a dressing gown and get straight into bed, staying there for an hour so that you work up a good sweat.

Drink between one and two cups of horsetail tea* while you are taking your sitz bath. Drink the tea slowly, one sip at a time.

Horsetail Tea
Drink two cups of horsetail tea* in the course of the day, taking care to sip it slowly.

Nettle Tea
Drink up to four cups of nettle tea* in the course of the day, taking care to sip it slowly.

Speedwell Tea
Drink one cup of speedwell tea in the evening before going to sleep, taking care to sip it slowly.

URINE (retention of)

Bedstraw Tea
Drink two or three cups of bedstraw tea* in the course of the day, taking care to sip it slowly.

Chamomile Wine
Pour 2 pt (1 l) of dry white wine into a saucepan and add four heaping teaspoonfuls of chamomile. Heat the wine up gently and remove it from the heat just before it comes to the boil. Let the chamomile steep for ten minutes before straining the wine into a glass bottle. Take two glasses of this wine every day, one in the morning after breakfast and the other in the evening after supper. Don't drink it too cold.

Deadnettle Tea
Drink one cup of deadnettle tea* every day after breakfast, taking care to sip it slowly.

Horsetail Vapor Baths
Place a bowl containing four teaspoonfuls of horsetail on the floor and pour in 2 pt (1 l) of hot water. Put on a robe, squat over the bowl and let the horsetail vapors act on your bladder for ten minutes.

You can also strain off the horsetail and use it in warm compresses. Wrap it up in a clean linen cloth and apply it to your bladder.

Nettle Tea
Drink up to four cups of nettle tea* during the day, taking care to sip it slowly.

Thyme Tea
Drink two cups of thyme tea during the day, taking care to sip it slowly.

UTERUS (diseases of)

Bedstraw Tea
Bedstraw is a reliable remedy for disorders of the uterus. Drink between two and three cups of bedstraw tea* a day, taking care to sip it slowly.

Horsetail Tea
Horsetail helps to staunch bleeding, and this makes it a useful remedy for uterine hemorrhages. Use three heaping teaspoons of horsetail for each cup of tea. Pour on hot water and let the herbs steep for thirty seconds before straining them off. Drink one or two cups of this tea in the course of the day, taking care to sip it slowly.

Lady's Mantle Tea
Drink up to four cups of lady's mantle tea* in the course of the day, taking care to sip it slowly.

Mistletoe Tea
The ability of the mistletoe to normalize blood-pressure, no matter whether it is too high or too low, makes it a good remedy for disorders of the uterus and also for troublesome periods.

Drink two or three cups of mistletoe tea* in the course of the day, taking care to sip it slowly. It's a good idea to keep your day's supply in a pre-warmed thermos.

Shepherd's Purse Tea
Take one heaping teaspoonful of shepherd's purse for each cup of tea. Pour on hot water and let the herbs steep for half a minute before sieving them off. Drink two to three cups of shepherd's purse tea* a day, taking care to sip it slowly.

Shepherd's purse also helps to staunch bleeding, which makes it particularly useful for treating uterine hemorrhages.

Yarrow Sitz Baths
In some cases a single yarrow sitz bath* can be enough to effect a cure. The water should be just deep enough to cover your kidneys. Stay in the bath for twenty minutes, and don't dry yourself off when you get out; put on a robe and get straight into bed. Stay there for an hour so that you work up a good sweat.

Yarrow Tea
Drink two to three cups of yarrow tea* a day, taking care to sip it slowly.

UTERUS (prolapse of)

Lady's Mantle Tea
Drink four cups of lady's mantle tea* in the course of the day, taking care to sip it slowly.

Shepherd's Purse Tincture
Massage your abdomen with shepherd's purse tincture,* starting at the vagina and working upward.

Yarrow Sitz Baths
Take three yarrow sitz baths* every week. The water should be just deep enough to cover your kidneys. Stay in the bath for twenty minutes, and don't dry yourself off when you get out; put on a robe and get straight into bed. Stay there for an hour so that you work up a good sweat.

VASOCONSTRICTION

Nettle Baths
Vasoconstriction can be cured with the help of nettle baths. Soak some fresh stinging nettles (leaves and stems) in 1 gal (5 l) of cold water for twelve hours. Then heat up the infusion gently and pour it, with the nettles, into your bathwater. Stay in the bath for twenty minutes.

VIRUS INFECTIONS

Calendula Tea
Drink three cups of calendula tea* during the day, taking care to sip it slowly.

Nettle Tea
Drink four cups of nettle tea* in the course of the day, sipping it slowly.

5. Standard Herbal Recipes

When you come across as asterisk after a recipe in either Chapter 3 or Chapter 4, this is referring you to the standard recipes listed here. However, please note that the recipe for a particular tea, for example, may vary according to the application. *Always* follow the instructions given under the specific ailment in the two preceding chapters, especially regarding quantities and frequency of use.

Agrimony Tea
Use one heaping teaspoonful of agrimony for each cup of tea. Pour on hot water and let the herbs steep for thirty seconds before straining them off.

Arnica Tincture
Fill a glass bottle two-thirds full with arnica petals, pulling the petals away from the protective green calyces. Pour enough 38-40% grain alcohol into the bottle to cover the petals completely, and leave the bottle to stand in a warm place for at least two weeks before use. Then strain some of the tincture into smaller bottles, leaving the remainder in the large bottle with the petals. You can then top up the bottle with some more alcohol. (Do not top it up more than once.)

Arnica tincture from the chemist's is usually made with 75% alcohol, and you should dilute it before use with an equal measure of cooled boiled water. The undiluted tincture is slightly corrosive, and can cause skin inflammations and lesions. Do not use on broken skin.

Bedstraw Tea
Use one heaping teaspoonful of bedstraw for each cup of tea. Pour on hot water and let the herbs steep for thirty seconds before straining them off.

Bedstraw Wash
Pour 1 pt (½ l) of hot water into a bowl containing two heaping teaspoonfuls of bedstraw and let it stand for thirty seconds before straining it.

Butterbur Root Tea
Use one level teaspoonful of butterbur root for each cup of tea and soak it in a cupful of cold water for twelve hours. Then heat up the infusion gently and strain it.

Calamus Root Bath
Soak 8 oz (200g) of calamus root in 1 gal (5 l) of cold water for twelve hours, then heat up the infusion gently and strain it into your bathwater.

Calamus Root Tea
Soak one level teaspoonful of calamus root in a cupful of cold water for twelve hours, then heat up the infusion gently and strain it.

Calendula Ointment
Unless other quantities are given, melt 8 oz (250g) of pure lard in a saucepan and add a generous handful of calendula leaves, flowers and stems. Bring the mixture to the boil, stirring it well, simmer briefly, then remove it from the heat. Put a lid on the saucepan and leave it to cool overnight. Then heat the contents up again gently until the fat is liquid enough to pass through a clean piece of muslin. Strain the mixture through the muslin, making sure that all the juice from the calendula is pressed through into the lard. The ointment can then be transferred to screw-top jars and should be stored in the refrigerator.

Calendula Tea
Use one heaping teaspoonful of calendula flowers for each cup of tea. Pour on hot water and let the flowers steep for thirty seconds before straining them off.

Calendula Tincture
Fill a glass bottle with calendula flowers and add enough 38-40% grain alcohol to cover them completely. Seal the bottle and leave it to stand in a warm place for at least two weeks before use.

Cedar Tincture
Fill a glass bottle with washed, finely-chopped cedar leaves and add enough 38-40% grain alcohol to cover them completely. Seal the bottle and leave it to stand in a warm place for at least two weeks.

Celandine Tea
Use one heaped teaspoonful of celandine for each cup of tea. Pour on hot water and let the herbs steep for thirty seconds before straining them off.

Chamomile Oil
Fill a glass bottle with freshly picked chamomile flowers and add enough oil to cover them completely. Seal the bottle and leave it to stand in a warm place for three weeks.

Chamomile Rinse
Pour 2 pt (1 l) of hot water into a bowl containing

a handful of chamomile flowers and let them steep for thirty seconds before straining them off.

Chamomile Tea
Use one heaping teaspoonful of chamomile for each cup of tea. Pour on hot water and let the herbs steep for thirty seconds before straining them off.

Chamomile Wash
Pour 2 pt (1 l) of hot water into a bowl containing a handful of chamomile flowers and let them steep for thirty seconds before straining them off.

Club Moss Tea
Use one level teaspoonful of club moss for each cup of tea. Pour on hot water and let the herbs steep for thirty seconds before straining them off.

Coltsfoot Tea
Use one heaping teaspoonful of coltsfoot leaves and flowers for each cup of tea. Pour on hot water and let the herbs steep for thirty seconds before straining them off.

Comfrey Root Tea
Use two heaping teaspoonfuls of finely-chopped comfrey roots for each cup of tea and soak them in a cupful of cold water for twelve hours. Then heat up the infusion gently and strain it.

Comfrey Root Tincture
Take enough comfrey roots to fill the glass bottle you are going to use, then wash them carefully under running water, scrubbing them with a brush. Chop the roots up finely and put them in a glass bottle. Add enough 38-40% grain alcohol to cover the roots completely. Seal the bottle and leave the tincture to stand in a warm place for at least two weeks before use.

Cow Parsnip Tea
Use one heaping teaspoonful of finely-chopped cow parsnip leaves for each cup of tea. Pour on hot water and let the herbs steep for thirty seconds before straining them off.

Cowslip Tea
Use one heaping teaspoonful of cowslips for each cup of tea. Pour on hot water and let the herbs steep for thirty seconds before straining them off.

Cowslip Root Tea
Use one heaping teaspoonful of cowslip root for each cup of tea. Pour on hot water and let the herbs steep for thirty seconds before straining them off.

Cranesbill Tincture
Fill a glass bottle with washed, finely-chopped cranesbill flowers, leaves and stems and cover them completely with 38-40% grain alcohol. Seal the bottle and leave it to stand in a warm place for at least two weeks.

Dandelion Root Tea
Steep a heaping teaspoonful of dandelion root in ½ pt (¼ l) of cold water for twelve hours. Then heat the infusion up gently and strain it.

Deadnettle Tea
Use one heaping teaspoonful of dead nettles for each cup of tea. Pour on hot water and let the herbs steep for thirty seconds before straining them off.

Golden Rod Tea
Use one heaping teaspoonful of golden rod for each cup of tea. Pour on hot water and let the herbs steep for thirty seconds before straining them off.

Hawthorn Tea
Use one heaping teaspoonful of hawthorn leaves and blossoms for each cup of tea. Pour on hot water and let the herbs steep for thirty seconds before straining them off.

Hawthorn Tincture
Fill a glass bottle with equal parts of freshly-picked hawthorn blossoms and berries and add enough 38-40% grain alcohol to cover them completely. Seal the bottle and leave the tincture to stand in a warm place for at least two weeks before use.

Horsetail Sitz Bath
Soak 4 oz (100g) of horsetail in 1 gal (5 l) of cold water for twelve hours. Then heat up the infusion gently and strain it into your bathwater.

Horsetail Tea
Use one heaping teaspoonful of horsetail for each cup of tea. Pour on hot water and let the herbs steep for thirty seconds before straining them off.

Horsetail Wash
Pour 2 pt (1 l) of hot water into a bowl containing four heaping teaspoonfuls of horsetail and let the infusion stand for thirty seconds before straining it.

Knotgrass Tea
Use one heaping teaspoonful of knotgrass for each cup of tea. Pour on hot water and let the herbs steep for thirty seconds before straining them off.

Lady's Mantle Tea

Use one heaping teaspoonful of lady's mantle for each cup of tea. Pour on hot water and let the herbs steep for thirty seconds before straining them off.

Maize Tassel Tea

Use one heaping teaspoonful of finely-chopped maize tassels for each cup of tea. Pour on hot water and let the herbs steep for thirty seconds before straining them off.

Mallow Tea

Soak a heaping teaspoonful of mallow in a cupful of cold water for twelve hours. Then heat up the infusion gently and strain it.

Mallow Wash

Soak two generous handfuls of mallow in 1 gal (5 l) of cold water for twelve hours. Then heat the infusion up slowly and strain it.

Marjoram Oil

Fill a glass bottle with marjoram and add sufficient oil to cover the herbs completely. Seal the bottle and leave the oil to stand in a warm place for three weeks before use.

Meadowsweet Tea

Use one heaping teaspoonful of meadowsweet flowers for each cup of tea. Pour on hot water and let the herbs steep for thirty seconds before straining them off.

Meadowsweet Tincture

Fill a glass bottle with freshly-picked meadowsweet flowers and add enough 38-40% grain alcohol to cover them completely. Seal the bottle and leave the tincture to stand in a warm place for at least two weeks before use.

Mistletoe Tea

Use one heaping teaspoonful of mistletoe for each cup of tea. Soak the mistletoe in a cupful of cold water for twelve hours, then heat the infusion up gently and strain it. Be sure no berries are present — Mistletoe berries are poisonous.

Nettle Bath

Soak a bucketful of fresh stinging nettle leaves and stems or 8 oz (200g) of dried nettles in cold water for twelve hours. Then heat up the infusion gently and strain it into your bathwater.

Nettle Footbath

Soak some fresh stinging nettle stems an leaves in 1 gal (5 l) of cold water. Then heat up the infusion gently.

Nettle Root Tincture

Fill a glass bottle with washed, finely-chopped spring or autumn stinging nettle roots and add enough 38-40% grain alcohol to cover them completely. Seal the bottle and leave it to stand in a warm place for at least two weeks.

Nettle Tea

Use one heaping teaspoonful of finely-chopped stinging nettles for each cup of tea. Pour on hot water and let the herbs steep for thirty seconds before straining them off.

Ointment

Use the quantities of herbs and lard indicated. Bring the mixture to the boil, simmer briefly, stirring it well, and then remove it from the heat. Put a lid on the saucepan and leave it to cool overnight. Then reheat the lard gently until it is liquid enough to pass through a clean piece of muslin. Strain the mixture through the muslin, making sure that all the juice from the herbs is pressed through the cloth into the lard. The ointment can then be transferred to screw-top jars and should be stored in the refrigerator.

Plantain Tea

Use one heaping teaspoonful of plantain leaves for each cup of tea. Pour on hot water and let the herbs steep for thirty seconds before straining them off.

Plantain and Thyme Tea

Dissolve a teaspoonful of brown sugar in a cupful of cold water, add a slice of lemon and bring to the boil. Then remove the pan from the heat and add a heaping teaspoonful of equal parts of Plantain and thyme. Let the herbs steep for thirty seconds before straining them off.

Ramsons (Broad-leaved Garlic) Tincture

Fill a glass bottle with finely-chopped ramsons leaves and bulbs and add enough 38-40% grain alcohol to cover them completely. Seal the bottle and leave the tincture to stand in a warm place for at least two weeks before use.

Ramsons (Broad-leaved Garlic) Wine

Put ½ pt (¼ l) of dry white wine in a saucepan and add a handful of fresh, finely-chopped ramsons leaves. Bring the wine to the boil briefly, then remove it from the heat, strain it and, if you wish, add a little honey.

Raspberry Leaf Tea

Use one heaping teaspoonful of freshly-picked, finely-chopped raspberry leaves for each cup of tea. Pour on hot water and let the herbs steep for thirty seconds before straining them off.

Sage Tea

Use one heaping teaspoonful of sage for each cup of tea. Pour on hot water and let the herbs steep for thirty seconds before straining them off.

St John's Wort Oil

Fill a glass bottle loosely with St John's wort flowers and add enough oil to cover them completely. Leave the sealed bottle to stand in a warm place for at least three weeks, until the oil turns a reddish color. Then strain the oil through a piece of muslin, pressing the flowers firmly so that none of their juice is lost. Store in small, dark glass bottles.

St John's Wort Sitz Bath

Soak a bucketful of St John's wort leaves, flowers and stems, or 4 oz (100g) of dried St John's wort, in cold water for twelve hours. Then heat up the infusion gently and strain it into your bathwater.

St John's Wort Tea

Use one heaping teaspoonful of St John's wort for each cup of tea. Pour on hot water and let the herbs steep for thirty seconds before straining them off.

Shepherd's Purse Tea

Use one heaping teaspoonful of shepherd's purse for each cup of tea. Pour on hot water and let the herbs steep for thirty seconds before straining them off.

Shepherd's Purse Tincture

Fill a glass bottle with freshly-picked, washed and finely-chopped shepherd's purse and add enough 38-40% grain alcohol to cover the herbs completely. Seal the bottle and leave the tincture to stand in a warm place for at least two weeks before use.

Sorrel Tea

Use one heaping teaspoonful of fresh, finely-chopped common sorrel leaves for each cup of tea. Pour on hot water and let the herbs steep for thirty seconds before straining them off.

Speedwell Tea

Use one heaping teaspoonful of speedwell for each cup of tea. Pour on hot water and let the herbs steep for thirty seconds before straining them off.

Speedwell Tincture

Fill a glass bottle with two generous handfuls of finely-chopped flowering speedwell and cover them with 2 pt (1 l) of 38-40% grain alcohol. Seal the bottle and leave the tincture to stand in a warm place for at least two weeks before use.

Swedish Bitters

½ oz (10g) aloe (or gentian root, or powdered wormwood if no aloe is available), ½ oz (10g) angelica root, ¼ oz (5g) carline root, ½ oz (10g) manna, ¼ oz (5g) myrrh, ½ oz (10g) natural camphor, ½ oz (10g) rhubarb root, 1 pinch saffron, ½ oz (10g) senna leaves, ½ oz (10g) *Theriak venezian*, ½ oz (10g) zedoary.

Place the above ingredients in a large glass bottle and add 2½ pt (1.5 l) of 38-40% grain alcohol. Seal the bottle and leave it to stand in a warm place for a minimum of two weeks, shaking it vigorously each day. For everyday use you can strain off some of the tincture into small bottles, which should be kept in a cool, dark place. The longer Swedish bitters are left to stand, the more potent they become.

Thyme Bath

Soak a good bucketful of fresh thyme, or 8 oz (200g) of dried thyme, in cold water for twelve hours. (A smaller quantity is sufficient for children: vary the amount to suit their constitution.) When the twelve hours are up, heat the infusion gently, then strain it into the bathwater.

Thyme Oil

Fill a glass bottle with freshly-picked thyme flowers and add enough oil to cover them completely. Seal the bottle and leave it to stand in a warm place for three weeks before using the oil.

Thyme Tea

Use one heaping teaspoonful of thyme for each cup of tea. Pour on hot water and let the herbs steep for thirty seconds before straining them off.

Walnut Leaf Tea

Use one heaping teaspoonful of walnut leaves for each cup of tea. Pour on hot water and let the herbs steep for thirty seconds before straining them off.

Walnut Leaf Wash

Steep two heaping teaspoonfuls of finely-chopped walnut leaves in 1 pt (½ l) of hot water for thirty seconds, and then strain off the leaves.

Wild Chicory Tea

Use one heaping teaspoonful of wild chicory for each cup of tea. Pour on hot water and let the herbs steep for thirty seconds before straining them off.

Wild Chicory Root Tea

Use one heaping teaspoonful of wild chicory root for each cup of tea and soak it in a cupful of cold water for twelve hours. Then heat up the infusion gently and strain it.

Willow-Herb Tea

Use one heaping teaspoonful of small-flowered willow-herb for each cup of tea. Pour on hot water and let the herbs steep for thirty seconds before straining them off.

Yarrow Sitz Bath

Soak 4 oz (100g) of yarrow (use all parts of the plant) in 1 gal (5 l) of cold water for twelve hours, then heat up the infusion gently and strain it into your bathwater.

Yarrow Tea

Use one heaping teaspoonful of yarrow for each cup of tea. Pour on hot water and let the herbs steep for thirty seconds before straining them off.

Yarrow Tincture

Fill a glass bottle with freshly-picked yarrow flowers and add enough 38-40% grain alcohol to cover them completely. Seal the bottle and leave the tincture to stand in a warm place for at least two weeks before using it.

Remedy and Plant Index

Therapeutic Index